Quit Lit Book for Women

CRAFTED BY SKRIUWER

Copyright © 2024 by Skriuwer.

All rights reserved. No part of this book may be used or reproduced in any form whatsoever without written permission except in the case of brief quotations in critical articles or reviews.

For more information, contact : **kontakt@skriuwer.com** (www.skriuwer.com)

TABLE OF CONTENTS

CHAPTER 1: UNDERSTANDING THE URGE TO PLEASE

- *How early life lessons can lead to people pleasing*
- *Spotting the signs of putting others first all the time*
- *Why this pattern might harm both your peace and relationships*

CHAPTER 2: RECOGNIZING HOW PLEASING OTHERS AFFECTS YOUR LIFE

- *Ways constant pleasing impacts work, family, and friendships*
- *Uncovering hidden costs like stress, worry, and lost identity*
- *Seeing when to change the pattern to protect your own well-being*

CHAPTER 3: BASIC STEPS FOR SETTING CLEAR LINES

- *What clear lines (boundaries) are and why they matter*
- *Common fears that block you from saying no*
- *Practical methods to protect your time and energy*

CHAPTER 4: HIDDEN PATTERNS THAT KEEP PEOPLE PLEASING

- *Discovering deep-rooted beliefs that push you to comply*
- *Replacing old habits of seeking approval*
- *Learning to spot triggers that pull you into people pleasing*

CHAPTER 5: LETTING GO OF OLD HABITS

- *Recognizing which habits keep you stuck and why*
- *Strategies to replace automatic yes with balanced choices*
- *Handling discomfort when you start changing your behavior*

CHAPTER 6: THE IMPORTANCE OF TRUTHFULNESS

- *Why honest communication is key to breaking people pleasing*
- *Differentiating truth from harshness or rudeness*
- *Learning to speak openly without guilt or fear*

CHAPTER 7: HANDLING WORRY AND NERVES

- *How anxiety shows up when you stand up for yourself*
- *Simple steps to calm a racing mind*
- *Turning worry into a sign that guides wiser decisions*

CHAPTER 8: BUILDING FRESH WAYS OF BEHAVING

- *Turning new insights into steady, daily habits*
- *Recognizing and avoiding slip-ups that drag you back*
- *Using routine and small goals to keep you on track*

CHAPTER 9: STRENGTHENING WHO YOU ARE

- *Finding your personal likes, values, and identity*
- *Trusting your own voice instead of outside praise*
- *Breaking free from fear of disapproval through self-awareness*

CHAPTER 10: FINDING PEOPLE WHO SUPPORT YOU

- *Why supportive relationships are vital for lasting change*
- *Identifying friends or groups that encourage your growth*
- *Handling negative people who resist your new habits*

CHAPTER 11: DEALING WITH GUILT AND SHAME

- *Understanding the difference between guilt (action) and shame (identity)*
- *How these feelings trap you in the pleasing cycle*
- *Practical ways to question and weaken them over time*

CHAPTER 12: BREAKING FREE FROM THE NEED TO BE PERFECT

- How perfectionism ties to people pleasing and approval-seeking
- Accepting "good enough" and learning from slip-ups
- Balancing high standards with self-compassion

CHAPTER 13: MAKING GOALS FOR REAL CHANGE

- Why specific, clear goals drive growth
- Structuring goals that push you without overwhelming you
- Tracking progress and adjusting plans to stay motivated

CHAPTER 14: METHODS TO HANDLE STRESS

- Spotting triggers that cause tension in your daily life
- Quick fixes (breathing, grounding) vs. long-term stress relief
- Protecting yourself from overload so you can hold your boundaries

CHAPTER 15: CARING FOR YOUR EMOTIONAL HEALTH

- Allowing and naming your feelings without judgment
- Building inner support systems through self-compassion
- Keeping emotional boundaries so you do not absorb others' problems

CHAPTER 16: STANDING FIRM IN DISAGREEMENTS

- Why conflict can be healthy and normal
- Steps to handle pushback or criticism calmly
- Avoiding extremes of aggression or retreating into fear

CHAPTER 17: GROWING MORE SELF-CONFIDENT

- Recognizing and replacing negative self-talk
- Taking on challenges to build inner trust
- Accepting praise and success without feeling awkward

CHAPTER 18: MOVING AHEAD WITH YOUR OWN DECISIONS

- *Separating your true desires from others' expectations*
- *Managing fear of making a "wrong" choice*
- *Standing by your decisions even when people disagree*

CHAPTER 19: PUTTING SELF-CARE INTO ACTION

- *Designing daily or weekly self-care routines that fit your life*
- *Handling guilt or pushback when you put yourself first*
- *Adjusting and protecting your self-care habits over time*

CHAPTER 20: CLAIMING YOUR PERSONAL POWER

- *Combining all lessons to live free from people pleasing*
- *Owning your worth and choices without losing kindness*
- *Maintaining healthy habits and relationships for lasting growth*

Chapter 1: The Reality of Drinking for Women

Women often face many demands each day. There can be pressure from work, family, and friends. In many cases, alcohol becomes part of daily life. Some women might have a glass of wine in the evening to calm their minds. Others might meet coworkers for drinks after a tough day. Still, others might feel the need to keep up with social expectations. Over time, these habits can become serious problems. This chapter looks at the real impact of alcohol on women's bodies and lives. The goal is to share facts that many do not realize until it is too late.

1.1 A Look at Current Trends

In many places, women are drinking more than they did years ago. Different surveys show that the number of women who drink regularly has climbed. There are reasons for this rise. One reason might be that women have more freedom than in past generations. Another reason could be that alcohol is easy to get. People see ads on TV, on billboards, or even on social media. Alcohol is sold in grocery stores, restaurants, and convenience shops. The barrier to buying it is very low.

Some marketing also targets women directly. You might see products named in a cute way to appeal to women. Or you may see bright, colorful packaging on wine bottles. Some ads show a woman relaxing with a drink in a bubble bath. These images can plant the idea that wine or cocktails are normal parts of a balanced lifestyle. This pushes the idea that women can handle more and more drinks.

At the same time, there are more stresses in many women's lives. Some juggle full-time jobs and full-time roles at home. Others deal with single parenthood. The pull to drink can feel strong. A woman may think, "I deserve this break," or "This is the only time for me to feel at ease." This mindset is not always voiced out loud, but it lingers in the back of many minds.

1.2 Unique Body Chemistry

Women's bodies are different from men's bodies. This is not a good thing or a bad thing. It is simply science. Women tend to have less total body water, which means alcohol remains more concentrated in their bloodstream. Women also have different levels of certain enzymes. These enzymes help the body break down alcohol. With lower levels, women's bodies process alcohol at a slower rate. This can lead to stronger effects in the short term and more serious damage in the long term.

Over time, regular drinking can harm women's livers. The liver is the main organ that processes alcohol. If it is asked to do too much, it wears down faster. This can lead to scarring of the liver, known as cirrhosis. Women can develop liver damage with lower amounts of alcohol compared to men.

Drinking can also affect a woman's hormones. Hormones play a big role in monthly cycles, mood changes, and stress management. Too much alcohol can throw these hormones off balance. This can lead to problems such as irregular cycles, stronger mood swings, or issues getting enough good-quality sleep.

1.3 The Hidden Impact on Health

Many women do not realize that regular drinking can lead to many long-term health problems. There is the risk of certain cancers, including breast cancer. Research shows that even small amounts of alcohol can raise breast cancer risk over time. There is also the matter of heart health. Some people believe a small glass of wine helps the heart. This might not be true for everyone. The bigger risk may come from the daily strain alcohol puts on the body.

Another concern is bone health. Women already face changes in bone density as they get older. Drinking can speed up bone loss, making bones weaker. This can lead to a higher chance of fractures. It might not happen right away, but years of regular drinking can add to bone issues.

Blood sugar problems can also arise. Alcohol can affect how the body handles sugar. If a woman is already at risk for diabetes, drinking may push her closer to that diagnosis. Blood pressure can also rise with frequent drinking. Some women find themselves on medication later in life because their bodies could not handle the extra burden placed by alcohol.

1.4 Everyday Life Problems

Aside from health problems, regular drinking can cause everyday issues. For example, missing work or showing up late because of a hangover can harm job stability. Or, some women might find they cannot function well in the morning, which makes their routines much harder. Those who have children may struggle to be fully present, leading to guilt or frustration.

A woman might also notice that her personal relationships suffer. Drinking can lead to fights with a partner or tension with family members. Trust can be broken if a person's behavior changes when they drink. A woman might promise her child or spouse that she would cut back, only to fall back into old habits a few days later. This can lead to shame and self-doubt.

Another factor is money. Alcohol can be expensive. A bottle of wine here or a cocktail there adds up quickly. Over weeks, months, or years, the amount of money spent can become a serious financial issue. This can lead to stress or arguments at home. Bills might go unpaid, or there may be less money for other needs. Yet, the person keeps buying alcohol because of the urge they feel.

1.5 Myths That Cloud Judgment

Many women come across myths that make them think drinking is not a big deal. One myth is that "a glass of wine at night is good for you." While one small glass of red wine might have some benefits for certain people, there is no hard rule that it is beneficial for all. Another myth is that "women can handle their alcohol just as well as men." Physically, this is often not the case. As noted before, women's bodies process alcohol differently.

Some women see alcohol as a reward or a sign of independence. You might hear someone say, "I'm a busy woman, so I deserve a drink." This can be a tricky path. Once you start pairing the idea of reward with alcohol, it can be easy to drink more often. You might say, "I got through Monday—time for a drink," or, "It's Friday, let's celebrate." And so on. Before long, you find that it's happening daily.

Another myth is that "if I keep it to just weekends, it's fine." Weekend drinking can still lead to problems. Some women only drink on Fridays or Saturdays, but they binge (have many drinks in a short time). This can harm the body just as much, if not more, than having a smaller amount each day. Also, binge drinking can lead to risky behavior, such as driving while impaired or making unsafe decisions.

1.6 Silence and Stigma

There is often an unspoken rule in many social circles: do not speak about your drinking problems. Women might fear being judged if they admit they are struggling. They might worry that others will see them as weak or irresponsible. Some women keep their concerns hidden from their closest friends. This silence can make the problem worse, because without talking about it, there is little chance to get advice or support.

In some cultures, there is the idea that a "proper" woman should not drink heavily. So, if a woman does find herself drinking too much, she might be afraid to come clean. She could feel that she is failing as a wife, mother, daughter, or friend. This shame leads her to hide the bottles or lie about how much she has had.

This secrecy also makes it harder to get medical help. Some women feel nervous telling a doctor how much they really drink. They might give a lower number, thinking it sounds more "acceptable." As a result, a doctor might not spot warning signs in blood tests or see the need to talk about treatment options. This can delay care until the problem becomes severe.

1.7 Real-Life Examples

1. **Anna** is a 35-year-old mother who works in an office. She started having a glass of wine after work to relax. Over a few years, that glass turned into half a bottle each night. She did not think it was a problem because it helped her calm down. Eventually, she noticed her kids' homework was not being checked thoroughly, and she was oversleeping. After her partner commented on her mood changes, she realized her drinking was affecting the whole family.
2. **Maria** is a 28-year-old professional who loves going out with friends. She typically limits herself to weekends, but she drinks a lot in those two nights. She often blackouts or forgets large parts of the evening. She used

to laugh it off, but after losing her phone multiple times, she began to worry. She also found random bruises and had no idea how she got them.
3. **Lisa** is a 42-year-old single woman who drinks several cocktails when she feels stressed. She justifies it by saying she has no partner or kids, so no one is harmed. Yet, she struggles with finances due to how much she spends on these cocktails. She also has missed out on career advancement because her work performance has dipped.

These examples show different ways that alcohol can creep into a woman's life. Each person's situation is unique, but they share a common thread: alcohol is creating trouble that builds over time.

1.8 Why It Is Hard to Quit

Quitting alcohol is not easy for many reasons. One reason is the physical side. If a woman has been drinking heavily for a while, her body might feel sick if she suddenly stops. This can show up as shaking hands, headaches, nausea, or anxiety. Some women also have trouble sleeping when they first quit. These symptoms can make it harder to stick to the plan of not drinking.

Another reason is the emotional side. A woman may have built a strong link between drinking and feeling calm or happy. Without alcohol, she might feel bored, stressed, or restless. If there is no plan for managing these feelings, it is easy to give in and reach for a drink. Also, if her social circle drinks often, she might feel left out if she does not join them. Fear of being the odd one out can push her back to drinking.

A third reason is that many women see no immediate harm. They might say, "I only have a few drinks, it's not that bad." But the damage can be slow and steady. It can remain under the surface for a long time, only to show up one day in a health crisis or a big event that jars everyone around them.

1.9 Short-Term vs. Long-Term Consequences

It is useful to separate the short-term and long-term effects. In the short term, alcohol can affect motor skills, judgment, and mood. This can lead to falls, car accidents, or saying things you regret. It can harm relationships or job performance. Some women might notice they become more sad or anxious the next day because alcohol disrupts the balance of brain chemicals.

In the long term, there is the risk of serious damage to organs, higher cancer risk, and mental health issues. Long-term drinking can lead to depression and anxiety that become harder to treat. It can also create tension in the home that does not easily go away. Children can be affected, too, especially if they see their mother's behavior shift drastically after a certain time of day or night.

1.10 Breaking the Pattern

Understanding the reality of drinking is the first step. Many women might read about these facts and see themselves in one or more examples. The next step is to decide what to do. Real change can begin when a woman admits that alcohol is causing her problems. From there, she can start to learn about resources, support groups, or medical help. She can look for healthier ways to handle stress, discover new methods to pass the time, and find emotional support that does not involve drinking.

This is not an instant fix. It might take time and patience. But many women find that once they confront the truth about how alcohol affects their bodies, minds, and relationships, they gain a drive to stop. They see that the short-term relief from a drink is not worth the long-term harm. Instead, they look for better ways to live.

1.11 Key Points to Remember

- Women's bodies do not break down alcohol the same way as men's bodies.
- Regular drinking can cause serious health issues, including higher risk for certain cancers, liver damage, and bone problems.
- Alcohol can harm relationships, job performance, finances, and self-worth.
- Myths about "healthy" amounts of wine or the idea that "women can handle it" can be misleading.
- Silence and stigma often keep women from seeking help.
- Awareness is the first step to making a positive change.

Chapter 2: Early Lessons and Influences

Many people start learning about alcohol before they ever take a sip. You might see it at family gatherings, on TV shows, or in commercials. You might notice a parent or older sibling drinking. Over time, these early lessons build a foundation for how you view alcohol. In this chapter, we explore how these lessons shape future behaviors. We also uncover how you can change what you learned in the past.

2.1 Family Modeling

One of the most direct ways to learn about alcohol is by watching family members. A child may see her mother having wine with dinner or her father drinking beer after work. Sometimes, the family has a casual attitude. They might say, "It's just an adult drink, no big deal." Other times, there might be strict rules, like "No one touches alcohol until they are 21." Or there might be conflict if one parent disapproves of the other's drinking.

A young girl might see a mother who drinks to cope with stress. If the mother never talks about her reasons, the child might assume that this is just how grown-ups handle problems. She might file that lesson away: "When life is stressful, open a bottle of wine." Years later, she might do the same thing without thinking much about it.

Some families use alcohol in a celebratory way, offering a toast for every achievement or special day. Even if the word "celebrate" is not used, the act of lifting a glass is still there, marking happy events with alcohol. Over time, the child learns that good times and alcohol belong together. When she grows up, she may keep this habit, feeling that no event is complete without a drink.

2.2 Cultural and Social Norms

Beyond the family home, there are cultural and social norms that shape how a girl sees alcohol. Certain communities may frown upon women who drink, while others may accept it freely. Some regions might have traditions that involve spirits or local brews, passing these practices down through generations. A woman might grow up around a culture that ties certain drinks to festivals, gatherings, or important rites.

In modern society, you also have the impact of social media. People post pictures of fancy cocktails or craft beers. They might make jokes about how they cannot get through Monday without coffee in the morning and wine at night. Memes often show that it is normal to rely on alcohol to handle daily life. Over time, these messages can blur the line between casual use and dependence.

It is also common to see strong advertising. Even if some words are avoided, the basic message is often that alcohol leads to a good time. Some ads show groups of women laughing and having fun, each holding a drink. If a young girl sees this image repeated often, she might decide that is what grown-up friendship looks like. Later on, she might feel odd if she does not have a drink in her hand when socializing.

2.3 Messages from Friends and Peers

When you get older and start spending more time with friends, their views on drinking can shape your own. In high school or college, peer pressure can be a big factor. Some teens hold parties where alcohol is present. Girls might be teased if they do not join in. Or they might be told, "Don't be boring." This can plant a seed that being fun means drinking.

In adulthood, peer pressure can still exist, though it might look different. Friends might say, "Let's grab a few drinks after work," or, "We're having a girls' night out—don't skip it." It might feel natural to go along, even if you are not in the mood for alcohol. Over time, this can become a regular habit that is hard to break.

Some women fear losing friendships if they stop drinking. They may worry that their friends will think less of them or leave them out of activities. This fear can be deep, especially if the social group is tight-knit and gatherings always include alcohol. Even if no one is forcing them, the subtle pressure is still there.

2.4 Media Portrayals

Television shows, movies, and books often show alcohol in certain ways. You might see a stressed mother who turns to a glass of wine once the kids are asleep. Or a single woman who finishes a rough day with a cocktail on her couch. These images look normal, so viewers might start thinking, "That's just part of life." Over time, it can shift public attitudes.

There are also programs where heavy drinking is shown as comedic. Characters might get drunk and do silly things. The audience laughs. If you watch these programs regularly, you might start to believe that getting drunk is just part of being funny or having a wild time. The damage or risks are rarely highlighted.

On the other hand, some shows do hint at the dark side of alcohol. But even then, it might be glamorized if the character is seen as edgy or troubled in a way that viewers admire. This can give confusing messages. A viewer might think, "Sure, she has issues, but she's also the most interesting character." In reality, there is little that is interesting about feeling sick, missing work, or hurting loved ones due to alcohol.

2.5 Personal Events and Milestones

Early lessons do not only come from watching others. Personal events in your own life can shape your relationship with alcohol. For instance, some teens have their first drink at a high school party. If the experience was positive and they felt included, they might repeat it. If it was negative, such as getting sick or being scolded by parents, they might avoid it for a while. But the memory stays.

College years can be a time when many women drink more heavily. They might see it as a rite of passage. If they have older friends who are partying, they might join to be part of the crowd. These experiences can lay the groundwork for how they use alcohol as adults. If heavy drinking was normal in college, they might keep that pattern after they graduate.

Big life changes can also influence how you see alcohol. If you moved to a new city for a job, you might use drinking as a way to meet people. Or if you started a stressful career, you might find yourself reaching for a glass each evening to take the edge off. Over time, these habits can become automatic.

2.6 Why Early Influences Matter

You might wonder why it is important to look back at these early experiences. The reason is that many women do not realize how these old lessons still shape them. You might think, "That was years ago. I'm a different person now." But the brain often holds onto these early rules. If you learned that "alcohol is the fastest way to relax," you might still use that tactic whenever stress hits.

These hidden beliefs can be strong. They guide day-to-day choices, even if you do not fully notice. By looking at your early influences, you can spot where your viewpoints about alcohol began. This can help you see that some of your beliefs may not be true or helpful anymore. This step can lead to a new way of thinking.

2.7 Unlearning What You Were Taught

Unlearning these old lessons is possible. It starts with awareness. Take a moment to think about your earliest memories of alcohol. Were your parents or family members big drinkers? Did you grow up in a culture where women never touched alcohol? Or one where it was offered freely at every meal? Did your friends tease anyone who did not drink?

Once you have a clear picture, ask yourself if these lessons are helping you now or holding you back. Maybe your mother's habit of wine after work seemed normal to you as a child, but now you see it as a path that led you to develop the same pattern. Or maybe your father always joked that a man can handle his drink, and you took that belief and tried to prove you could handle it just as well.

It helps to replace these old lessons with new facts. For example, you might have grown up thinking alcohol is the best way to reduce stress. Now, you can learn about other ways, such as taking a walk, listening to music, or talking with a trusted friend. By repeating these new habits, you teach your brain that there are better choices. Over time, your view on alcohol can change.

2.8 Breaking Generational Cycles

Some families have patterns that stretch across generations. A grandmother might have had alcohol problems, which led her child (your mother or father) to adopt certain habits. This can move down the line to you. Breaking a generational cycle is not easy, but it can be done. The first step is to admit that this cycle exists. The next step is to decide you do not want to continue it.

You might notice that talking about alcohol was taboo in your family. No one brought it up, even though everyone knew a certain uncle or aunt had a problem. By naming the issue and seeking help, you set a new standard. Younger relatives might see you as an example and think, "We don't have to pretend everything is fine. We can do things differently."

Breaking these cycles can also bring healing to family relationships. If you decide to stop drinking, it might prompt other relatives to rethink their habits. This does not always happen, but sometimes seeing one person step forward can inspire others.

2.9 The Role of Guilt and Shame

Sometimes, when women look back at their early lessons, they feel guilty for having believed something for so long. Or they might feel shame about how much they have been drinking. It is helpful to remember that no one is born knowing all the facts. People learn from their environment. If your environment taught you to drink as a coping method, it is not your fault that you followed that teaching. What matters now is what you decide to do about it.

Guilt can be a strong emotion. It might cause a woman to shut down and refuse to face her past. Shame can make her hide her habits even more. The aim is not to blame yourself for your early lessons but to see them for what they are—old scripts that might no longer serve you.

2.10 Changing the Narrative

It is useful to think of your relationship with alcohol as a story you have been telling yourself. Maybe the story is, "I'm just a social drinker. This is normal." Or,

"I come from a family of drinkers, so this is just who I am." You can change that story.

Start by writing down the beliefs that come to mind when you think of alcohol. Do you believe it helps you relax? Do you believe everyone around you drinks, so you must too? Next, ask yourself if those beliefs are always true. Can you find any times when you relaxed without alcohol? Do you really need to drink to fit in, or is it that you just do not have practice socializing without alcohol?

This process might feel odd at first, but it can help shift your perspective. Instead of seeing drinking as the only path, you begin to see other roads. You might find that you like certain calming activities, such as reading a mystery novel or knitting. The key is to keep trying new approaches.

2.11 External vs. Internal Motivation

When changing lessons learned long ago, you need to tap into your own motivations. There are two main types of motivation: external and internal. External motivation might come from a spouse who says, "Quit drinking or I'll leave," or from a doctor who says, "Your liver tests are bad; you need to stop." These outside factors can be strong, but internal motivation is usually more sustainable. Internal motivation is driven by your personal choice and your desire to be healthy, happy, or more at peace.

If you rely only on external motivation, you may stop drinking out of fear or because you feel forced. That might work in the short term, but it can lead to resentment later. If you find a deep internal reason—such as wanting to live longer to see your children grow up, or wanting to improve your own self-esteem—that can power you forward for the long haul. Reflect on why quitting is important to you, personally. That will help you break free from the old lessons that hold you back.

2.12 Setting Boundaries with Influences

Once you decide to challenge your early lessons, you might need to set boundaries. If your old friend group always goes to bars, you might have to limit how often you join them. Or if family gatherings are always filled with booze, you might choose to arrive late, leave early, or bring your own non-alcoholic drinks. Some people worry about seeming rude, but your health is more important than meeting everyone else's expectations.

Boundaries can also be internal. For instance, you might set a rule: "No drinks in the house." By making alcohol less accessible, you help yourself avoid temptation. If you used to watch TV shows that made you want to drink, you can switch to different content. These small steps can add up and make a big difference over time.

2.13 Using Past Lessons for Good

Early lessons do not have to be negative. You might recall certain family members or friends who avoided alcohol and seemed perfectly content. Or you might have had a teacher who explained the dangers of underage drinking. Perhaps these lessons did not stick at the time, but you can revisit them now. If you remember good advice you were given, try to act on it. Sometimes, a small piece of wisdom from the past can be a powerful force in the present.

If you have kids or younger relatives, you can use your experiences to teach them. Show them that alcohol is not a requirement for fun or stress relief. Talk openly about what you wish you had known sooner. These honest chats can help them form healthier habits from the start.

2.14 A Fresh Start

Each day is a chance to rewrite the lessons you learned. If you spent decades thinking that a drink after work is the only way to relax, remind yourself that there are other ways. If you believed you had to drink to fit in, challenge that assumption. Try going to a social event and ordering a non-alcoholic beverage. You might feel awkward at first, but many people will not even notice. They might be too busy with their own conversations to care about what is in your glass.

Over time, these new patterns become your normal. You train your brain to see alcohol as unnecessary. You might still be around people who drink, but it will not have the same hold on you as before.

2.15 Key Points to Carry Forward

1. **Family influence**: How parents or siblings used alcohol can shape your own habits.
2. **Social and cultural norms**: These can plant strong beliefs about how women should act with alcohol.
3. **Peer pressure**: Friends can influence your decisions, both in younger years and as an adult.
4. **Media messages**: TV, movies, and ads can make alcohol appear normal or harmless.
5. **Unlearning and rewriting**: You can choose to reject old lessons that no longer serve you.
6. **Boundaries**: Changing your environment and social routines can help you stick to healthier habits.
7. **Internal motivation**: Tapping into your personal reasons for cutting out alcohol will keep you strong.

By looking at the source of your beliefs about alcohol, you gain the power to shape a new mindset. These early influences do not have to dictate your life forever. In the next chapters, we will continue exploring how to recognize triggers, manage stress, and set up better supports. Before we move on, take a moment to reflect on what you learned in these first two chapters. Think about which early lessons apply to you and how you can start challenging them today.

Chapter 3: Social Pressures and Myths

3.1 Understanding the Social Scene

When many women think about alcohol, social events often come to mind. These events might be nights out with friends, happy hour gatherings, or family get-togethers. You see people holding glasses, chatting, and seeming relaxed. It is easy to feel that having a drink is the "normal" thing to do. This can create a strong push, especially if you are trying to stop drinking. You might wonder if people will think you are odd for not joining them.

Social pressure is not always direct. Sometimes, no one tells you, "You have to drink." Instead, it is a feeling that you might not fit in if you do not have a glass in your hand. This sense of belonging is powerful. Many women fear that if they do not go along with the group, they might lose friends or harm their connections at work. But there are ways to see through these pressures. It begins by recognizing that a lot of them rest on myths.

3.2 The Myth of "Everyone Drinks"

One strong myth is that "everyone drinks." You might see social media posts showing your peers with cocktails. You might notice colleagues mentioning weekend gatherings. All of this can give the impression that no one stays sober anymore. In reality, many people do not drink at all or only do so on special occasions. You just might not notice them because they do not make a big announcement about it.

Researchers have found that there are plenty of groups who choose not to drink. They might have health reasons, personal beliefs, or simply do not like how it makes them feel. Some folks might attend the same parties but only sip a soda or a glass of water. This is often overlooked because our attention is drawn to those who do have alcoholic drinks.

The key point is that not everybody is drinking. If you decide not to drink, you are not alone. You are part of a large, although sometimes quieter, group that is also steering clear of alcohol. By reminding yourself of this fact, you can lessen the feeling that you are missing out.

3.3 Media and Hollywood Myths

Television and movies often show women bonding over drinks. This can create the idea that a close friendship requires sharing a bottle of wine. You might see characters in a show gather at a local bar after a tough day, giving each other advice while sipping cocktails. Over time, these images can stick in your mind. You might come to believe that deep connections only form when people drink together.

However, this is a created image meant to sell a storyline. If you look behind the scenes, you will find that real bonds can form in many ways. Some women go hiking, some join book clubs, and others meet at coffee shops. Sure, there might be movies that show those things, but they are less attention-grabbing than a scene with colorful cocktails. The fact remains: you can have meaningful friendships without alcohol.

3.4 The "Drink to Fit In" Mentality

Many women fear that they will stand out if they are the only one not drinking. They might worry about being teased. They might even worry about making others feel judged. The idea is that if you do not have a drink in your hand, people will think you are dull or antisocial. This notion can push even the most reluctant drinker to join in.

But let's look at it logically. If your friends truly care about you, they will accept your choice. They might ask questions at first, but good friends typically want you to be healthy and at ease. Also, many times, people are busy enjoying their own evening. They might not even notice what is in your glass. If someone does push you to drink, that might say more about their comfort level than about your choices. Sometimes, folks who are uneasy about their own habits try to get everyone to join them to feel less guilty.

3.5 The Myth That Alcohol Is Harmless in Moderation

A common statement is: "Alcohol in moderation is good for you." Some people cite a study that suggests a small glass of red wine helps the heart. Others claim that moderate drinking promotes relaxation. While it is true that small amounts of some drinks may have certain properties, it can be risky to generalize. The definition of "moderation" varies from person to person, and women's bodies react differently than men's.

Also, the benefits some people talk about might be met by other means, like improving diet or staying active. You do not need wine to keep your heart healthy if you follow other good health routines. In truth, many health experts say that even a small daily intake of alcohol can raise certain risks for women, such as breast cancer. These facts often get lost in the swirl of social messages.

3.6 The Myth of "Liquid Courage"

It is common to hear people call alcohol "liquid courage." The idea is that drinking a bit can help a shy person open up. Some women might feel they cannot talk to new people at a gathering unless they have a drink to calm their nerves. However, this mindset can become a crutch. Over time, you may forget how to socialize without some help from alcohol.

Real self-assurance does not come from a glass. It comes from building skills and feeling comfortable in your own skin. Relying on alcohol can hide the underlying anxiety for a while, but it usually does not fix it. Once the effect wears off, the worry often returns, sometimes stronger than before. The result is a cycle where you keep needing "liquid courage" to function in social settings. Breaking this cycle can open the door to real personal growth.

3.7 Pressure from Friends and Family

Sometimes the push to drink is strongest from people you know well. Friends might say, "Come on, just one more," or "Don't be a buzzkill." Family members might say, "Our family always has wine with dinner," or "You're no fun without a drink." These comments can hurt more than passing remarks from strangers because they come from those close to you.

One approach to this issue is planning your response in advance. You can say something simple and calm, like, "I'm not drinking tonight. I'm trying something new." If they press you for details, you can repeat your statement or change the topic. It might feel odd at first, but this approach keeps you from getting drawn into a long debate. Sometimes, people push because they want to see if you are serious. Standing firm can show them you mean it.

Another strategy is to discuss your decision privately with people who matter. For instance, if your sister always nudges you to have a cocktail, you might sit down and say, "I have decided to stop drinking. Please help me by not offering me any." If she truly cares, she will respect that request. If she refuses, it might be time to set firmer boundaries for your well-being.

3.8 Pressure in the Workplace

In many work environments, drinking is part of socializing. Your boss might hold a Friday event at a local bar. Coworkers might invite you to join them for a "team-building" beer. Turning these invites down can be challenging if you worry that it might affect your professional image. You might fear that saying no makes you look unfriendly or not committed to team bonding.

However, it is worth considering your overall goals. If your workplace respects personal choices, you can join the event but order a non-alcoholic drink. It is often the mingling that matters, not the alcohol. If anyone asks, you can say, "I am fine with my soft drink," and keep the conversation flowing about work topics or shared interests.

In some workplaces, you might face a culture where alcohol is deeply ingrained. This can happen in fields where entertaining clients is normal. In that case, you may want to talk to a mentor or HR representative about how to manage it. Sometimes, employers understand that not everyone can or wants to drink, and they will support your decision. If they do not, it might prompt you to consider if that environment is healthy for you in the long run.

3.9 Bar Culture and Restaurant Norms

When you go out with friends, you might gather at restaurants, bars, or clubs. Many of these places expect patrons to buy drinks. Some even have specials like "ladies' night" to draw in more customers. The music is loud, the lights are dim, and the mood seems tied to having a glass in your hand. If you do not order alcohol, you might get a look from the waiter or bartender.

But realize that bars and restaurants are businesses. Their aim is to sell items, including alcoholic drinks. Of course, they want to encourage you to buy another round. That does not mean you have to comply. You have the right to order water, tea, or a non-alcoholic alternative. Some establishments now offer "mocktails" (drinks made without any alcohol) that are flavorful. If the place does not have these options on the menu, you can politely ask for a soda with lime or something similar.

One tip is to hold your glass just like everyone else does. If you do not make a big deal about it, many people will not notice you are sipping something alcohol-free. This can help you blend in if you want to avoid questions. Over time, you may feel more relaxed about standing out, but in the early stages of quitting, this tactic can be helpful.

3.10 Online Groups and Peer Influence

In today's world, online communities can also play a role in social pressure. You might join groups for women that share memes about "wine o'clock" or "mommy juice." People joke about needing wine to get through the day. While these jokes might seem harmless at first, they can normalize daily drinking. If you express a desire to stop, you might feel odd or even unwelcome.

It can help to seek online groups that support sobriety or healthy living. There are forums and social media pages where people encourage each other to stay alcohol-free. Reading their experiences can remind you that you are not alone. You can also share your struggles and triumphs with others who understand. This can balance out the more casual groups that treat drinking as a standard part of life.

3.11 The Myth That Women Should Drink Specific Alcohol

Some ads and even some social circles push the idea that certain drinks are "feminine." Examples might include sweet wines, fruity cocktails, or rose-colored beverages. They might suggest that beer or whiskey are "manly" drinks. These notions try to pigeonhole women into certain roles. They also make it seem that a stylish woman must have a glass of pink bubbly to match her outfit.

In truth, there is no rule about who "should" drink which beverage. Marketing experts created these images to sell more products. Real people have varied tastes, and some do not like the taste of alcohol at all. Reminding yourself of this fact can free you from the idea that you must choose a certain drink to be seen as ladylike or trendy. If you do not want any alcohol, you can pick a different option without feeling you are breaking a social code.

3.12 Breaking Free from Pressures

If you want to stop drinking, standing up to these social pressures is key. That does not mean you must avoid all social events. Instead, you can approach them with a plan:

1. **Decide your reason for not drinking**: Be clear on why you are making this choice. It might be for health, finances, or personal goals. Keeping your reason in mind helps you stay firm when faced with questions.
2. **Practice your response**: Sometimes, people will ask why you are not having alcohol. Rehearse a simple statement, such as, "I am focusing on my health," or "I'm cutting back right now."
3. **Bring a friend who supports you**: If you feel outnumbered, invite a friend who respects your choice. Having someone on your side can ease the tension.
4. **Know your exit plan**: If an event becomes too awkward, it is okay to leave early. You do not owe anyone a long stay if you feel uncomfortable.
5. **Reward yourself in other ways**: Some people find they have extra money saved from not buying drinks. Use that for something you enjoy, like a new book or a relaxing activity. This helps reinforce your decision.

3.13 Challenge the Myths

Many of the social pressures rest on myths that "everyone drinks," "it's harmless," and "you need it to have fun." Look at these myths closely:

- **"Everyone is doing it."** We covered that this is not true. Many people do not drink, but they may not broadcast it.
- **"It is harmless in small amounts."** Even small amounts can affect you, especially over time. Women's bodies are more sensitive to alcohol's effects than men's.
- **"Alcohol is needed to be sociable."** That is an illusion. People have built strong friendships through sports, hobbies, volunteer work, and other shared interests without alcohol.

By spotting these myths for what they are, you can reduce their hold on you. This step might seem small, but it is powerful. Once you question the validity of a myth, it no longer seems as logical or unshakable.

3.14 Building Real Confidence

One of the big reasons people give in to social pressures is a lack of confidence. It is not easy to be the one who says, "No thanks, I'm not drinking tonight." But the more you practice, the more self-assured you will become. Think of it as building a new skill. Each time you refuse a drink with grace, you gain a bit more self-trust.

You might also notice that saying no to alcohol makes you feel better the next day. You are clear-headed, not hungover or tired. You might have extra time to do things you enjoy. Over time, this pattern can lead to a stronger sense of self. You realize you do not need to follow the crowd to be happy or accepted.

3.15 Key Points to Take Forward

- Social pressure can come from friends, family, media, and even your workplace.
- Myths about alcohol are widespread: that everyone drinks, that small amounts are always fine, that it is a must for fun.
- You can learn to handle events without feeling like you need a glass in your hand.
- True friends will respect your choice to stay sober. Those who push you might be covering their own worries.
- Confidence grows each time you stick to your plan.

Moving on, the next chapter will look at the medical facts and unique health risks women face when they drink. Knowing these facts can strengthen your resolve to challenge social myths. It is one thing to suspect that drinking might be bad for you, but it is another to see the specific health reasons why it can be risky. Use the tips in this chapter to handle social situations in a way that aligns with your goals and well-being.

Chapter 4: Medical Facts and Unique Health Risks

4.1 How Alcohol Moves Through the Body

When a person drinks alcohol, it passes through the mouth and into the stomach. A bit is absorbed in the stomach, but most moves into the small intestine. From there, it enters the bloodstream. Once it is in the blood, it travels to different organs, including the liver, brain, and heart. The liver is in charge of breaking it down into less harmful substances, but it can only process a small amount per hour. If someone drinks more than the liver can handle, alcohol remains in the bloodstream longer, affecting the brain and other parts of the body.

Women tend to have less body water than men, so alcohol does not get diluted as much. This means the same amount of alcohol can result in a higher blood alcohol level for a woman compared to a man of a similar weight. Women also have lower levels of certain enzymes involved in breaking down alcohol. This is why women can experience stronger effects from smaller amounts of alcohol.

4.2 The Role of Hormones

Hormones play a big role in women's health. They affect mood, energy levels, and reproductive function. Alcohol can disrupt the natural hormone balance, leading to multiple issues. For instance, it can throw off the monthly cycle. Some women find their periods become irregular or more painful when they drink regularly. Hormone problems can also worsen mood swings and lead to tiredness.

In addition, alcohol can increase estrogen levels in some women. High estrogen is linked with certain types of cancer, including breast cancer. While not every woman will have the same exact reaction, it is important to know that alcohol can raise the odds of hormone-related problems.

4.3 Impact on Reproductive Health

Women who are pregnant or trying to become pregnant face special risks with alcohol. Drinking during pregnancy can affect the unborn baby's growth. It can lead to physical or mental challenges for the child. Even moderate drinking can raise these risks. Health experts often advise that women who are pregnant or may become pregnant avoid alcohol completely.

There are also concerns about fertility. Some women have trouble getting pregnant because of underlying health conditions. Alcohol can make it harder by affecting hormone levels, ovulation, and overall health. While many factors go into fertility, cutting out or reducing alcohol is one step that might improve the chances of conceiving. It also supports a healthier environment for the baby if a pregnancy occurs.

4.4 Bone Density

Women face an increased chance of bone density loss as they age, especially after certain stages in life. Chronic drinking can accelerate this process. Alcohol interferes with the body's ability to absorb calcium and vitamin D, both of which are important for keeping bones strong. Over the long term, this can lead to thinner bones, a higher chance of fractures, and conditions like osteoporosis.

Once bone density is lost, it is hard to rebuild. This is why prevention is key. Making sure you get enough nutrients, doing weight-bearing exercise, and keeping alcohol intake low (or zero) can help protect bones. If you are already concerned about your bone health, consider talking to a medical professional about a bone density scan. This can give you a clear picture of any risks.

4.5 Effects on the Heart

Some people claim that red wine is good for the heart. In reality, the research on this is mixed. There may be elements in red wine that can support heart health, but the alcohol itself can do more harm than good, especially for women. Drinking can raise blood pressure, increase certain fats in the blood, and contribute to weight gain. Over time, these factors can strain the heart.

Also, women who drink heavily have a higher risk of cardiomyopathy (a disease of the heart muscle) and other heart problems. If there are heart conditions in your family, you might want to be extra careful about alcohol. Avoiding it could reduce your chances of developing serious heart issues down the road.

4.6 Liver Health

The liver's job is to filter out toxins, including alcohol. When you drink, the liver works hard to process it. Over time, this can lead to inflammation of the liver.

Women can develop alcoholic hepatitis or cirrhosis after fewer drinks over a shorter period compared to men. Cirrhosis is a serious condition where healthy liver tissue is replaced by scar tissue. This scarring can make it difficult for the liver to function well.

Once cirrhosis sets in, it cannot be reversed. This is why paying attention to liver health is crucial. Early signs might include fatigue, nausea, or pain in the upper right part of the abdomen. Sometimes, there are no symptoms until the damage is severe. Regular checkups and blood tests can help catch problems early, but the best defense is cutting back on alcohol or quitting altogether.

4.7 Brain and Nervous System

Alcohol can affect the brain in both short-term and long-term ways. Right away, you might notice issues with coordination, slurred speech, or slowed reaction time. These effects can lead to accidents and injuries. But the bigger concern is what happens over years of drinking. Long-term use can change the structure of the brain and impact how it communicates with the rest of the body.

Women's brains may be more vulnerable to alcohol-related harm. Some studies indicate that women can develop memory problems or cognitive decline faster than men who drink the same amounts. It might also heighten the risk of depression, anxiety, or other mental health problems, which can then feed the desire to drink again. This can become a cycle that is hard to break without professional help.

4.8 Connection to Cancers

When people think of alcohol and cancer, they often focus on liver cancer. While that is a valid worry, there is a strong link between alcohol and other cancers as well. Women who drink regularly have a higher risk of breast cancer. Alcohol can also be linked to mouth, throat, and digestive tract cancers. Even a moderate intake can raise these odds over time.

These findings come from many years of medical studies. The reason is that alcohol can change how cells function and grow. It can interfere with DNA repair, making cells more likely to become cancerous. Reducing or avoiding alcohol can lower these risks, though it does not guarantee safety from cancer. Other factors like family history also play a part. However, cutting back can remove one significant risk from your life.

4.9 Diabetes Risk

Type 2 diabetes is a growing concern for many adults. It happens when the body cannot use insulin effectively. Alcohol can affect blood sugar levels, sometimes making them drop too low (hypoglycemia), especially if you drink on an empty stomach. For some people, drinking leads to weight gain, which is another risk factor for diabetes.

Women who already have prediabetes or a family history of diabetes should pay attention to their alcohol use. Reducing or eliminating it can help stabilize blood sugar and possibly keep prediabetes from turning into full diabetes. If you already have diabetes, drinking can make managing it more complicated, as alcohol may interfere with medications and throw off your meal schedules.

4.10 Skin and Appearance

While health is usually the main focus, appearance also matters to many women. Alcohol can have a direct effect on the skin. It can lead to dehydration, causing dryness and dullness. Some women experience facial redness due to widened blood vessels. Over time, heavy drinking can worsen issues like acne or rosacea.

Drinking can also disrupt your sleep, which affects skin renewal. When you do not get good rest, it often shows on your face in the form of dark circles or a tired look. By cutting out alcohol, you might notice a brighter complexion and healthier-looking hair and nails. This benefit might seem superficial, but it can boost self-esteem in a big way.

4.11 Effects on Mood Disorders

Women are more likely than men to experience certain mood disorders, such as depression or anxiety. Alcohol can worsen these conditions. While some people feel a brief sense of relief when they drink, the aftereffects often include heightened sadness, irritability, or nervousness. This happens because alcohol changes the balance of chemicals in the brain and can lead to withdrawal symptoms once it wears off.

If you already deal with a mood disorder, alcohol can make medications less effective. It might also mask the true nature of your symptoms, making it hard for doctors to assess your needs accurately. Cutting back on alcohol or quitting altogether can be a big help in improving your emotional well-being, even though it might feel hard at first.

4.12 Sleep Problems

A common myth is that alcohol helps a person sleep. While it might make you feel drowsy, it disrupts the normal sleep cycle. You might fall asleep quickly, but you are more likely to wake up after a few hours, unable to get restful sleep. You can also experience less of the deep stage of sleep that the body needs for healing and memory formation.

Women are more prone to sleep disturbances, especially during certain phases of life. If you add alcohol on top of that, it can cause even more issues. Over time, lack of quality rest can affect your mood, energy, and physical health. Quitting alcohol often leads to better sleep patterns, which can improve many other parts of daily life.

4.13 Alcohol and Prescription Drugs

Many women take prescription drugs for various health reasons—birth control, antidepressants, blood pressure medication, or diabetes medication, to name a few. Mixing alcohol with these medications can lead to serious problems. It can reduce the effectiveness of birth control, raise blood pressure, or cause extreme sedation.

Always read the labels on any medications you take. Many state clearly to avoid alcohol or to use caution. If you are not sure, ask your doctor or pharmacist. Keep in mind that some over-the-counter drugs, such as cold or allergy medicines, can also be affected by alcohol. These interactions can be dangerous, making it vital to stay informed and aware.

4.14 Long-Term Health Outlook

If you keep drinking over many years, the effects pile up. Small harms that do not seem serious at first can grow into major health troubles. This includes fatty liver disease, heart problems, or a higher cancer risk. Some women assume that they have time to cut back later, but the truth is that the damage can start earlier than you think.

The good news is that stopping or reducing alcohol use can often slow, halt, or even reverse some of the damage, depending on the condition. The body is resilient, and many organs can heal if they get the chance. By quitting now, you give yourself a better shot at a healthier future.

4.15 A Path Toward Better Health

After reading about these risks, you might feel worried or overwhelmed. That is normal. The point is not to scare you, but to show how alcohol can have many impacts on a woman's body. If you are trying to stop, these facts might help you stay motivated. You are not only reducing your cancer risk or helping your liver—you are also looking after your bones, heart, and mental state.

If you are unsure where to start, consider getting a checkup with a medical professional. You can explain that you are thinking about giving up or reducing alcohol. They might run tests to check your liver enzymes or talk to you about your risk factors. Having real data about your health can be eye-opening. It can also help you track your improvement over time if you stop drinking.

Tips to Support Better Health:

1. **Stay hydrated**: Drink plenty of water. This helps flush out toxins and keeps your organs in better shape.
2. **Add nutrients**: Eat a balanced diet with enough vitamins, minerals, protein, and healthy fats. Your body can heal faster if it gets the right fuel.
3. **Maintain activity**: Regular movement strengthens the heart and bones, and it also helps with mood regulation.
4. **Manage stress**: If you used alcohol to cope, find safer methods like breathing exercises, writing in a journal, or talking to a trusted friend.
5. **Get sleep**: Aim for a consistent bedtime and a relaxing routine. Proper rest is vital for physical and mental well-being.

Conclusion of Chapter 4

Women face unique health risks related to alcohol. The combination of body chemistry, hormone factors, and societal pressures can create a tricky path for those trying to manage or quit drinking. Yet, knowing these medical facts is a big step toward positive change. Once you see how many parts of your body and mind can be harmed by alcohol, it becomes clearer why quitting or cutting back can lead to real benefits.

Chapter 5: Family and Household Factors

5.1 Introduction: The Influence of the Household

One important part of a woman's decision to drink or not drink is her home life. The household includes partners, children, parents, or anyone else living under the same roof. What goes on inside these walls can either strengthen a woman's will to remain alcohol-free or lead her to keep drinking. In this chapter, we will look at the ways family members and daily routines can add pressure, create stress, or provide much-needed support.

The goal is to shine a light on how hidden patterns in the home might affect a woman's use of alcohol. Many people assume their personal choice to drink does not harm others. But alcohol misuse can shape the entire mood and atmosphere of a household. If you want to quit drinking, it is wise to check what is happening at home and how it might help or hurt your progress.

5.2 The Spouse or Partner Factor

If you have a spouse or partner, that person can be a key factor in your drinking habits. In some cases, a partner also drinks regularly. It could be that both of you use alcohol as a way to relax after a long day. When this happens, it can be tough for one person to quit if the other keeps drinking. You might feel left out or think that your partner does not support your goals.

On the other hand, a partner could be against alcohol. They might nag you or shame you about your drinking. Though they might have good intentions, their harsh approach can make it more difficult for you to quit. Feeling judged can cause resentment, which might drive you to keep drinking in secret. This leads to dishonesty in the relationship.

A healthy approach is for you and your partner to have an honest talk about the role of alcohol in your life. Explain why you want to quit. Ask for their understanding and, if possible, their help. They do not need to stop drinking completely if they do not want to, but it would be easier if they reduce how much they drink around you, at least in the early stages. Some partners are willing to try a "dry month" or reduce how much they keep in the house. This kind of teamwork can cut the temptation and make you feel supported.

If your partner also has a drinking problem, your decision to quit might create tension. Sometimes, people prefer to stay in denial rather than face the fact that their household environment feeds the habit. Be prepared for pushback if your partner is not ready to face their own drinking. Stay calm and focused on your own choice. You can offer resources or suggest that both of you get help together, but in the end, they have to make their own decisions. You can only control your own actions.

5.3 Effects on Children

Children are quick to notice patterns in the home. They observe when a parent comes home in a bad mood and heads straight for a glass of wine or a bottle of beer. They listen to arguments or see changes in mood caused by drinking. They might not fully understand the situation, but they sense tension in the air.

When a mother drinks often, children might feel neglected or confused. They might worry about how to help, or they might blame themselves. Some children act out at school because they are upset or stressed at home. Others become very quiet and withdrawn. Over time, children can develop their own harmful ideas about alcohol. They might believe that it is normal to use it for stress or that adults always come home and drink.

Quitting can improve your ability to be present for your children. You can have clear conversations, help them with homework, and take them to their activities without worrying about whether you are in the right frame of mind. It also sets an example of how to deal with problems. By choosing to face life without relying on a substance, you show them a healthier path. This can make a deep difference in the kind of adults they grow into.

If you find it hard to talk to your children about your decision to quit, you can start with simple statements. You might say, "I used to have a drink when I felt stressed, but now I'm learning other ways to handle stress." You do not have to share every detail if they are young. The main thing is to let them know it is not their fault and that you are taking steps to be better. This honesty can help them feel secure.

5.4 Household Routines and Habits

Daily routines play a big role in a woman's drinking habits. Maybe you always open a bottle of wine while cooking dinner. Or you sit down to watch TV at night with a drink in hand. These routines can become so ingrained that you do them without thinking. The physical home space can also matter. For instance, if you store alcohol in a visible spot, you will be reminded of it every time you walk by.

Changing small things in your routine can help. If you usually have a drink while making dinner, switch to a different activity. You might sip on a flavored water or herbal tea. You might also start dinner prep earlier so you are not as rushed, cutting down on your stress. If you are used to drinking while watching a show, consider picking up a book or doing a quick exercise routine during commercials.

It also helps to rearrange your home. If you keep alcohol in the fridge door, move it to a less noticeable place, or remove it from the house entirely if you can. This cuts down on visual triggers. You could also store healthy snacks or non-alcoholic drinks in easy reach. This way, when you feel the urge to do something with your hands or mouth, you have a better option close by.

5.5 Emotional Atmosphere: Stress, Conflict, and Resentment

The emotional atmosphere in a household can drive a woman to drink or stay sober. If the home is full of arguments or unresolved problems, it can feel overwhelming. A woman might think, "I need a drink just to get through this evening." Over time, these patterns deepen. The household becomes a place where negative feelings brew, and alcohol is used as a temporary escape.

One way to tackle this is to address conflicts head-on. If you and your partner or family members have constant disagreements, consider honest communication strategies. Set aside time when everyone is calm. Explain how certain actions or words make you feel. Listen to their side without interrupting. Sometimes, families find that writing down their concerns before talking can help avoid heated fights.

Therapy or counseling can also help if tensions run high. A trained counselor can teach healthy communication methods and help you spot harmful patterns. If you are working on quitting, a counselor can also guide you through the household changes that need to happen. It might feel strange at first, but many families find it worthwhile to invest in professional support.

5.6 Extended Family and Cultural Factors

Extended family members—such as grandparents, aunts, uncles—can affect your habits as well. Maybe there is a tradition in your extended family that always involves alcohol. You might feel pressure to keep that tradition alive. Or an older relative might say, "All the women in this family drink. It's just what we do." This can cause guilt or confusion when you decide to stop.

Boundaries can help here. If you know a certain family event always ends up with everyone drunk, you might choose not to attend, or at least leave before the heavy drinking starts. You might also speak to the host in advance, letting them know you will not be joining in with the drinks. This can be uncomfortable at first, but being upfront helps you avoid misunderstandings.

Cultural norms are also key. In some cultures, refusing an offered drink is seen as rude. You might face pushback if you say no. While it is important to respect your culture, it is also important to respect your health. You can politely decline and say something like, "I'm focusing on my health right now," or "I'm not drinking these days." Most people will eventually accept your choice if you stay calm and consistent.

5.7 Parenting Responsibilities and Guilt

Women who have children often face guilt when they realize their drinking habits might affect how they parent. You might look back at times you snapped at your kids because you were hungover or moody. This guilt can be very heavy. Some women respond to guilt by drinking more, trying to numb the feelings. It becomes a vicious loop.

The healthier way is to face that guilt, acknowledge it, and decide to act differently going forward. You cannot change the past, but you can make changes today. This might mean having a heartfelt talk with your kids, apologizing for times you were not at your best. It might involve seeking help from a counselor who can guide you in managing guilt. By choosing to be sober, you give your children a more stable environment. Over time, this will bring healing and build trust.

5.8 Shared Financial Burdens

Money is another household factor that can cause stress and lead to more drinking. Bills, mortgage, rent, and basic living costs can become a point of conflict if money is tight. Some women might try to handle stress by having a drink to relax. But alcohol costs add up, which can worsen the financial strain. This tension can lead to more arguments at home and create a negative spiral.

A good starting point is to sit down with your partner or a trusted family member and create a budget. See exactly how much is going toward alcohol. The numbers might be surprising. If you find that your spending on alcohol is taking away from savings or other needs, that realization can motivate you to quit. You can then channel that money into something more useful, like a family trip or an emergency fund. This shift can reduce money-related arguments and create a sense of relief for everyone.

5.9 Household Responsibilities

Think about all the tasks that must be done in a home: cooking, cleaning, grocery shopping, laundry, and so on. If you are the one doing most of these tasks, you might feel overworked. Some women use alcohol as a reward or a break from the never-ending chores. But once you decide to quit, it is worth re-examining how chores are divided. Could you ask your partner or older children to pitch in more?

If you feel supported at home with these tasks, you might be less inclined to seek a "break" in the form of a drink. Having a well-structured household can reduce stress levels. Write down all the chores, assign them to different family members, and set up a schedule. This might feel odd if you have been doing everything yourself. But remember, a more even workload can boost family harmony and take away some stress that triggers drinking.

5.10 Handling Visitors at Home

Sometimes, the household environment changes when visitors come by. Maybe your friend stops over in the evening, and your usual habit is to open a bottle of wine. Or your sister visits for the weekend, and you both tend to share drinks for fun. Changing these habits can be hard. You might worry that your visitor will be disappointed or think you are no longer fun.

Before they arrive, you can let them know you are not drinking. Suggest other activities or beverages. You might prepare a tasty non-alcoholic punch, buy sparkling water with fruit slices, or plan an outing that does not center on alcohol. The goal is to show that you can still be warm and welcoming without serving or drinking alcohol. True friends or relatives might need time to adjust, but they will likely come to respect your decision.

5.11 Broken Trust and How to Repair It

For women who have been drinking heavily for a while, there might be a history of broken trust in the home. You might have made promises to cut back but did not follow through. You might have hidden bottles or spent money without telling your spouse. These actions can cause a lot of pain in a relationship.

Repairing broken trust takes time. You can start by being honest about your goal to quit. Share your plan: maybe you are reading this book, going to a support group, or seeing a counselor. Then, follow through on what you say. Each day that you remain honest and sober adds a small brick back into the foundation of trust. If you slip up, admit it rather than hide it. Transparency is key.

You might need to give your family time to see that you really mean it this time. They may still be cautious or expect a relapse. Instead of taking offense, understand that they are protecting themselves from disappointment. Show them, through consistent actions, that you value their trust enough to stay on track. Over time, most loved ones start to believe in your changes.

5.12 Secrets and Enabling

In some households, there is a pattern of keeping secrets around alcohol. Maybe a spouse buys the alcohol and pretends not to notice how much you are drinking. Or a teenage child helps to hide the evidence because they do not want you to be upset. This is known as enabling. The family members might believe they are helping, but they are actually allowing the behavior to continue.

When you decide to quit, you need to break the secrecy. Ask family members not to buy alcohol for you. Ask them not to cover for you if you slip. If you are honest about what is happening, they might at first feel uneasy. But over time, they will see that open communication leads to genuine change. It also teaches them that they do not have to tiptoe around the issue anymore.

5.13 Creating a Positive Environment

It is easier to stop drinking when your home feels calm and supportive. You can take steps to make the environment brighter and more uplifting. Some people find that adding a few plants, opening windows for fresh air, or playing relaxing music can shift the mood in the house. Others put positive reminders or quotes on the fridge. These might be simple statements like, "I am free to choose a better life."

Encourage laughter and fun in the household that does not involve alcohol. Game nights, movie marathons, or family walks around the neighborhood can bring everyone together. When the focus moves away from drinking, you may find that you all bond in new ways. Over time, these positive moments can replace the old memories linked with alcohol. This helps form a new "normal" for the household.

5.14 Dealing with a Toxic Household

Sometimes, a woman's household is truly toxic. Perhaps the partner is abusive or other family members pressure her to drink. In these cases, quitting becomes more complicated because the environment itself is harmful. If you are in such a situation, consider seeking help beyond what a self-help book can provide. You might need to talk to a shelter, a counselor, or legal authorities if you face abuse.

It takes courage to admit that your home might not be safe. But trying to quit while in a toxic setting can be an uphill battle. Think about your well-being first. Reach out to hotlines or support services in your area. They can guide you on steps to find safety, which is often a needed step before successful long-term sobriety is possible.

5.15 Building Long-Term Strength

Once you create a healthier household, do not let your guard down. The decision to quit drinking might become easier, but life will still present challenges. Family members will go through ups and downs. Stressful events can happen unexpectedly. To stay strong, keep communication open, maintain or adjust household routines as needed, and seek outside help if problems arise.

You can also encourage a family culture of positive habits. This might include cooking nutritious meals together, setting weekly goals, or having everyone share something good about their day at dinner. By placing the focus on wellness and togetherness, you reduce the role that alcohol once played.

5.16 Conclusion of Chapter 5

Family and household factors have a big influence on a woman's drinking habits. A supportive environment can pave the way for a smoother transition to an alcohol-free life. But a hostile or stressful home can make quitting far more difficult. Awareness is the first step: look closely at your home life, your daily routines, and how your loved ones respond to your choice to quit. Once you pinpoint the stress points, you can make a plan to address them.

Chapter 6: Money Problems Linked to Alcohol

6.1 Introduction: The High Cost of Drinking

Drinking alcohol might seem like a small expense at first. You might pay for one bottle of wine here and a few cocktails there. But these costs add up. Many women are surprised when they tally their monthly or yearly spending on alcohol and related activities. Beyond the direct cost of drinks, there are indirect costs: missed work, health care expenses, and even accidents that can lead to big bills. This chapter looks at the financial toll alcohol can take and explores ways to handle money better once you stop drinking.

Managing money is already stressful for many people. When alcohol gets added to the picture, stress can double or triple. Some women try to ignore it, feeling they "need" that glass of wine or bottle of beer no matter the cost. But acknowledging the money aspect can be a powerful motivator to quit. Imagine what you could do with the extra funds once you remove alcohol from your budget. That alone might make you realize how drinking is draining your finances.

6.2 Daily or Weekly Spending

One of the simplest ways to see the impact on your wallet is to track daily or weekly spending. Let's say you buy a bottle of wine each night for ten dollars. That's seventy dollars a week. In a month, that's about three hundred dollars. Over a year, that's more than three thousand dollars. And that is just the direct cost of the alcohol itself.

If you usually go out to bars or restaurants, the total can be even higher. Cocktails at a bar might cost ten to fifteen dollars each, sometimes more. If you go out multiple times a week and have a few drinks each time, your monthly spending can skyrocket. Then factor in tips, transportation, or extra food you might order because you are drinking.

Some people do not realize how big a chunk of their paycheck is going toward alcohol. They might think, "It's only a few dollars here and there." But writing it down or using a budgeting app can reveal the truth. This is often a wake-up call. Not only do you see the total, but you also notice patterns in your spending—like drinking more on specific days of the week.

6.3 Hidden Costs: Health Care and Insurance

Beyond the direct spending on drinks, there are hidden costs linked to drinking. One major area is health care. If you develop liver problems, high blood pressure, or other conditions tied to alcohol, you could face medical bills for tests, hospital stays, or medications. Even if you have insurance, you might need to pay deductibles or co-pays.

In some cases, alcohol can contribute to accidents—like a slip or fall at home or a car crash if someone drives under the influence. These incidents might lead to emergency room visits, legal fees, or an increase in your insurance premiums. If you are cited for driving while intoxicated, you could face fines or the cost of a legal defense. Some people lose their driver's license, which impacts their ability to get to work or maintain a job.

Insurance companies also tend to charge higher rates if you have a history of alcohol-related health problems. This could affect not just health insurance, but life insurance or other policies. Over time, these hidden costs can add up to a large sum. Many women do not see this connection right away, but it becomes clear when they face unexpected bills.

6.4 Impact on Career and Income

Drinking can affect your ability to hold a steady job or earn promotions. If you are frequently hungover, your productivity can drop, and you may miss important deadlines or meetings. Over time, this can prevent you from advancing in your career, which limits your income potential. In severe cases, a person might even lose their job due to alcohol-related issues like tardiness or poor performance.

Even if you manage to keep your job, you might not be giving it your best effort. This can mean fewer opportunities for raises or bonuses. If you run your own business, a drinking habit can hurt your decision-making and leadership. You might make poor choices that cause the business to lose clients or revenue. These effects might not be immediate, but over months or years, they can become significant.

Some women might blame stress at work for their drinking, saying they need to unwind. But then the drinking itself creates more problems at the job. It becomes a cycle: stress at work leads to a drink, the drink leads to lower performance, which leads to more stress, and so on. Breaking this loop can help you regain focus and energy, which in turn can boost your career prospects.

6.5 Debt and Financial Anxiety

Many people carry some form of debt, such as credit cards, student loans, or car loans. Adding alcohol expenses to an already tight budget can deepen the debt. If you find yourself unable to pay bills on time because you spent extra money on drinks, late fees and interest charges might pile up. This can create a wave of financial anxiety that affects other parts of your life.

When a person is anxious about money, it can trigger more drinking as a form of escape. This is another loop that is tough to break if you are not aware of it. You might be so worried about how to pay rent or cover credit card bills that you reach for a drink to calm your nerves, but that drink costs money and leads to more guilt. Addressing the root of the problem—alcohol spending—can help break this cycle.

6.6 Social Spending and Peer Pressure

A lot of social events revolve around bars or outings where alcohol is served. If you are trying to keep up with friends who drink, you might feel pressure to spend money you do not have. Some women keep ordering rounds or fancy cocktails so they do not look "cheap." Others might feel guilty turning down a friend's suggestion to have one more drink. Before you know it, the bill is much larger than you expected.

By quitting, you take back control of your spending at social events. You can still go out if you choose, but you will not be dropping cash on multiple rounds of drinks. If you are worried about what friends will think, you can plan ahead. For example, if a friend suggests an expensive club, you can say, "Let's meet for lunch instead," or "I'm trying to save money, so how about a coffee shop?" True friends will respect your desire to be financially responsible.

6.7 Planning a New Budget

Once you decide to quit, it is helpful to sit down and create a fresh budget. Look at your income, your mandatory expenses (like rent or mortgage, utilities, food, transportation), and your discretionary expenses (like entertainment, clothes, and so on). You can now remove or greatly reduce the line item for alcohol. This might free up a noticeable chunk of money.

Decide what you want to do with those freed-up funds. It could go toward paying down debt, building an emergency savings account, or funding a hobby you enjoy. Some people find it empowering to see that what used to go toward alcohol can now be put to a more positive use. This might be the first time you feel you are taking real control of your money instead of letting old habits dictate your spending.

6.8 Future Goals and Dreams

Alcohol can be a roadblock to reaching bigger life goals. Perhaps you always wanted to take classes to upgrade your skills or go on a special trip with your family. But each month, the money set aside for that goal disappears in bar tabs or liquor store runs. By quitting, you can redirect those funds where they truly matter.

Write down some of your dreams, whether they are short-term or long-term. Maybe you want to start a small business one day. Or you might want to invest in real estate. Even if your goals are more modest, like buying a better car or fixing up your house, you will be surprised how much faster you can save when you cut out alcohol costs. This sense of progress can keep you motivated to stay sober.

6.9 Unexpected Savings in Other Areas

Quitting does not just save money on the alcohol itself. There are other ripple effects. For example, you might cook more meals at home instead of eating out (which often includes alcoholic drinks). Cooking at home can be cheaper and healthier. You might also spend less on late-night snacks or fast food, because many people who drink also end up buying convenience foods.

You might notice your healthcare costs go down in the long run, too. Fewer doctor visits, lower insurance premiums, and fewer prescription medications can all come from improved health after quitting. Even if you do not see a big drop right away, over the years these savings can be significant. It becomes one more reason to stay on track.

6.10 Handling Relapses and Financial Setbacks

It is possible you might slip and have a drink at some point, leading to unplanned spending again. Relapses happen, and they can bring guilt or frustration. This might also cause a small financial hit if you went overboard and spent money you could not spare. The key is to not let one setback destroy your entire plan.

A good approach is to have a plan for slip-ups. Set aside a little "miscellaneous" fund in your budget in case something goes off track. That way, you are not thrown into a panic if you overspend once. But do not treat this as permission to relapse regularly. Instead, see it as a safety net while you learn new habits.

If you do relapse, look at what triggered it. Was it stress, a celebration with friends, or boredom? Identifying the root cause can help you prevent it next time. Then, refocus on your financial goals. Remind yourself of what you are aiming for—paying off debt, saving for something important, or simply having financial peace of mind.

6.11 Building a New Relationship with Money

Many women have an uncomfortable relationship with money. They might feel guilty spending on themselves, or they might spend recklessly without a plan. Quitting alcohol can open the door to a healthier mindset about money. Instead of feeling powerless, you start making conscious choices.

One technique is to use a cash envelope system for discretionary spending. Put a set amount of cash in envelopes each month, labeled for different purposes like "Dining Out," "Clothes," or "Entertainment." Once an envelope is empty, you are done spending in that category until the next cycle. This method helps you see exactly where your money goes and prevents overspending.

Another strategy is to set small, measurable goals. For instance, "I will save fifty dollars a week for the next three months." Track your progress on a calendar or an app. As you see that amount build, you gain confidence. This sense of control can carry over into other parts of life, reminding you that you do not need alcohol to deal with stress or boredom.

6.12 Teaching Financial Responsibility to Children

If you have children, your decision to quit can teach them valuable lessons about money. You can talk openly (in an age-appropriate way) about how much money you used to spend on alcohol and how you are now using it for better things. Show them how you set goals, create a budget, and make choices to stick to that budget.

For example, if your child wants a toy, you can explain how you are saving up for it in the same way you are saving on alcohol expenses. You can say, "I used to spend money on wine, but now I'm putting that money aside for fun family activities." This not only strengthens your resolve but also instills good money habits in your children. They see first-hand that skipping unnecessary expenses can lead to bigger rewards.

6.13 Reclaiming Time and Effort

Quitting can also free up your time and energy. Drinking often leads to late nights out, extra time spent recovering from hangovers, or repeated trips to the store. By eliminating alcohol from your routine, you might notice you have more hours in the day to focus on productive tasks. This can indirectly help your finances as well.

With more energy and clarity, you might decide to pursue a side job or a small home-based business for extra income. Or you might put more effort into your main job, leading to promotions or recognition. All these actions can improve your money situation. The best part is that it does not feel forced, because you genuinely have more drive once you stop numbing yourself with alcohol.

6.14 Dealing with Social Events and Gifts

Some people spend a lot of money on drinks at social gatherings or buying bottles as gifts when they visit friends' houses. This pattern can strain your finances. Once you stop drinking, you might feel awkward showing up without a bottle of wine. But you can choose other thoughtful gifts: a nice plant, a box of specialty tea, or a homemade dessert. These items are often cheaper, and they do not push you into a drinking environment.

Your friends might even appreciate the variety, realizing they do not need to receive another bottle of wine they may not want. Over time, this can spread through your social circle, inspiring others to think differently about gift-giving and entertaining. All it takes is one person to suggest a change.

6.15 Using Financial Wins as Motivation

Seeing your bank balance grow can be a powerful motivator. Whenever you feel tempted, think about how you can spend that money in a better way. Maybe you can treat yourself to a relaxing massage, buy a comfortable new pair of shoes, or put money toward an online course to upgrade your skills. These rewards can reinforce the positive side of quitting.

It might help to keep a visual reminder. For instance, you can keep a jar where you place the cash you would have spent on alcohol each week. Watch the jar fill up. When you have a decent amount, use it for something meaningful or fun. This physical evidence can remind you of the financial benefits of saying no to alcohol. It can also be a way to involve your family, letting them see and celebrate the changes too.

6.16 Conclusion of Chapter 6

Alcohol can create serious money problems. Direct costs, hidden health care bills, and lost job opportunities can all eat away at a woman's financial stability. Stopping drinking not only improves health and family life—it can also free up funds for more important goals. By examining your spending, planning a new budget, and redirecting money toward positive uses, you can overcome the financial pitfalls that often go hand in hand with alcohol use.

This chapter showed how quitting can reduce debt, cut anxiety, and open doors to bigger dreams. Whether you want to fix your house, invest for the future, or simply stop living paycheck to paycheck, removing alcohol from your expenses can be a big step forward. Keep in mind that changing your money habits takes time and patience, just like changing any other habit. But once you see the benefits—both in your bank account and your overall peace of mind—you will likely feel even more determined to stay sober.

Chapter 7: Mental Health Concerns

7.1 Introduction: The Mind-Body Link

When a woman thinks about quitting alcohol, she often focuses on physical health or family issues. Yet, mental health is just as important. Drinking can affect mood, thoughts, and how a person feels about herself. It can also bring about strong emotions like sadness, anger, or shame. Many women do not realize how closely linked their mind and body are until they begin to see problems. This chapter looks at how alcohol use connects to mental health. It also shows ways to handle issues like anxiety, depression, or deep stress without relying on a drink.

7.2 How Alcohol Affects the Brain's Chemicals

The brain has chemicals that help control mood and behavior. Common ones include serotonin, dopamine, and GABA. These are not fancy words you need to memorize, but it helps to know they keep the brain in balance. When you drink, alcohol changes the levels of these chemicals. At first, you might feel calm or cheerful. That is because alcohol can raise dopamine levels briefly. However, once the effect wears off, dopamine and other chemicals can drop below normal levels. This makes you feel down or anxious.

If a person keeps drinking for a long time, the brain tries to adjust. It might reduce how much of these chemicals it makes on its own. That is why, over time, a woman might need more alcohol to get the same effect. When she stops drinking, she might feel jittery or depressed because her brain is not used to managing its own chemicals. Understanding this process helps explain why quitting can lead to intense moods at first.

7.3 Anxiety and Alcohol

Anxiety is a feeling of worry or fear that does not go away. It can show up as a racing heart, sweaty palms, or the sense that something bad is about to happen. Many women reach for alcohol to calm these feelings. For a short time, it might seem to help. However, once the alcohol wears off, anxiety often comes back stronger.

This pattern can lead to what some people call "rebound anxiety." In other words, the worry is even worse than before, which leads a person to drink again.

Over time, this cycle grows. A woman might not be able to handle daily tasks without alcohol because she fears that her anxiety will be too much. This is how drinking becomes tied to anxiety. When you quit, anxiety can spike at first, but there are better ways to manage it (more on that later in the chapter).

7.4 Depression and Low Mood

Depression is another common mental health concern linked to alcohol. People with depression may feel persistent sadness, lose interest in normal activities, or have trouble getting out of bed. While alcohol can momentarily numb emotional pain, it tends to worsen overall mood. Alcohol is a "downer" substance in the long run. It can sap energy and increase hopeless thoughts.

Women who are depressed might drink to forget their problems. Yet, drinking often leads to missing work, arguments with loved ones, or physical issues. These can pile on more guilt or sorrow, worsening depression. Quitting can be a big help, even if it feels hard at first. Without alcohol clouding the mind, a woman might be better able to seek real solutions for her low mood, like talking with a counselor or trying an antidepressant if a doctor suggests it.

7.5 Self-Esteem and Shame

Another mental health issue linked to alcohol is low self-esteem. Some women feel worthless or embarrassed when they think about how much they drink. They might see themselves as weak. This can turn into shame, which is the feeling that something is deeply wrong with who they are as a person. Shame can lead to hiding the problem, which then leads to more drinking.

Sometimes, shame comes from society or family. A woman might have grown up in a place where people say a "good" woman does not drink too much. If she does, she is labeled as irresponsible or immoral. This can force her to pretend everything is fine, never asking for help. Shame can also arise from repeated failed attempts to quit. She might think, "I tried before and I couldn't stop, so I must be hopeless."

Understanding that alcohol addiction is a health issue, not a moral flaw, is crucial. It is also helpful to see that shame does not have to be permanent. By learning better ways to handle stress, working on self-care, and reaching out for support, a woman can repair her sense of worth.

7.6 Panic Attacks and Sleep Problems

Women who drink might face panic attacks. These are sudden bursts of intense fear, often with physical symptoms like a racing heart, dizziness, or shaking. Alcohol disrupts the normal balance in the brain, so when the body is not getting the alcohol it is used to, it can trigger panic. This can happen at night or in the middle of an ordinary day. The experience can be scary.

Another issue is sleep disturbance. Many women say alcohol helps them fall asleep faster. But it actually disrupts the quality of sleep. The body never enters the deep stages of rest for long. This can lead to fatigue, irritability, and increased anxiety the next day. Breaking this cycle can help restore healthier sleep patterns and reduce panic episodes.

7.7 The Influence of Trauma

Trauma refers to events that severely shake a person. This could be anything from a past abusive relationship to a scary incident. Many women who have experienced trauma turn to alcohol as a form of self-medication. It dulls the memories or flashbacks for a while. Yet, the problems remain under the surface.

In fact, alcohol can make trauma symptoms worse over time. It can increase emotional numbness and keep a woman stuck in the past. Recovery from trauma often requires therapy or counseling that focuses on safety and coping methods. Quitting drinking is a key part of this process because it helps the brain start to heal. Once a woman is sober, she can engage more effectively with mental health support.

7.8 Understanding Co-Occurring Disorders

Sometimes a woman has both an alcohol problem and another mental health disorder. This is known as a "co-occurring disorder." For instance, she might have generalized anxiety disorder and also rely on alcohol. Or she might have bipolar disorder and binge drink. These conditions can fuel each other. A woman might need her anxiety medication adjusted because drinking weakens its effect, or she might skip therapy sessions because she is hungover.

Treating a co-occurring disorder often means addressing both problems at once. If a woman only treats her depression while ignoring her alcohol use, she might not improve. If she tries to quit drinking without looking at her underlying anxiety, she might relapse. Integrated care, where a mental health professional and possibly an addiction specialist work together, can lead to the best results.

7.9 The Path to Healing the Mind

Deciding to quit drinking is a big step toward better mental health. However, it is not a magic switch. A woman who has been relying on alcohol might suddenly feel raw emotions come flooding back. That can be tough at first. The key is to have a plan for dealing with these emotions. Here are some approaches:

1. **Talk Therapy**: This can be with a psychologist or counselor who helps you unpack your thoughts and feelings. You learn coping methods and healthier responses to stress.
2. **Group Support**: Some women find it helpful to join a group where they can talk openly about both mental health and addiction. Hearing others share similar experiences reduces feelings of isolation.
3. **Medication**: Under a doctor's care, some women benefit from medication for anxiety or depression. This does not mean you are weak; it just means you are using all available tools.
4. **Lifestyle Adjustments**: Regular exercise, good sleep, and balanced meals can support better mental health. These habits help the brain regulate its chemicals more effectively.

7.10 Stress Management Techniques

Stress is a normal part of life. But if a woman has been relying on alcohol to manage stress, she needs new methods. These can include:

- **Breathing Exercises**: Simple techniques like slow, deep breaths can calm the nervous system.
- **Progressive Muscle Relaxation**: Tensing and then relaxing groups of muscles can ease tension in the body.
- **Mindful Activities**: Using adult coloring books, easy crafts, or gentle stretching can give the mind a place to focus other than worry.
- **Short Walks**: A brief walk outdoors can help clear the head. Nature can have a soothing effect.

These methods might feel awkward at first, but with practice, they can become a steady way to handle stress without turning to alcohol.

7.11 Breaking the Isolation

One big factor in mental health is isolation. A woman who drinks might pull away from friends who do not drink as much. She may avoid family members who question her habits. Over time, she feels alone, even if she is surrounded by people. Loneliness can worsen depression and anxiety.

Quitting calls for rebuilding connections or forming new ones. That might include reaching out to a friend you have not spoken to in a while or joining a community group that does not revolve around alcohol. Human beings thrive on connection. Even if you are shy, finding a small group or a single person to share with can lift your spirits. Online support communities can also help if in-person contact is hard.

7.12 Handling Emotional Triggers

Emotional triggers are feelings that prompt a craving. For some women, it might be sadness. For others, anger or boredom. Recognizing these triggers is key to protecting your mental health. For instance, if you know that after a stressful argument you tend to reach for a drink, you can plan ahead. Maybe you will step outside for fresh air, do a quick writing exercise, or call a supportive friend instead.

Keeping a small notebook of triggers can help. Write down when you feel an urge to drink and what emotion or event sparked it. Over time, patterns emerge. You might see that fights with a partner trigger anger or that slow weekends trigger boredom. Then you can work on solutions for each situation. This process takes patience, but it is a strong step in safeguarding your mental health.

7.13 Building a Sense of Hope

Without hope, it is hard to stay sober. Many women fall into patterns of thinking that nothing will ever get better. Alcohol becomes a way to block out that hopeless feeling. Rebuilding hope involves setting small goals and noticing progress. For instance, maybe you manage five days without a drink and see a boost in your mood. Or you tackle a problem at work more clearly because your mind is not clouded.

Acknowledging these wins can raise optimism. You might still have bad days, but having evidence of good changes helps you push through. Some people keep a journal of small victories—like "I woke up today with more energy" or "I got through an argument without needing a drink." Over time, these notes remind you that growth is real.

7.14 Support from Loved Ones

If you have supportive family or friends, tell them about your mental health concerns. Explain that quitting is not just about the physical effects of alcohol, but also about how you feel inside. They might not fully understand at first, but most caring individuals will want to help. They can check in on you, ask how you are coping, or give you space if you need quiet time.

For women who do not have a strong support system at home, outside resources like counseling or community support groups are vital. You do not have to do this alone. Mental health issues can worsen when you feel you have no one to turn to.

7.15 Warning Signs that Help Is Needed

Sometimes, quitting can uncover deeper mental health problems. You might realize you have constant thoughts of harming yourself or that you cannot function at all without a drink. If this happens, do not wait. Reach out for professional help. Warning signs include:

- Thoughts of ending your life.
- Inability to get out of bed or do basic tasks.
- Hearing or seeing things that are not there.
- Severe panic attacks that make you feel like you cannot breathe.
- Complete breakdown in relationships due to your mental state.

Health experts or crisis lines can guide you to the right level of care. It might mean a short hospital stay or a more intense form of therapy. This is not a failure; it is a responsible choice to protect your life.

7.16 Long-Term Emotional Maintenance

Once you have handled the immediate mental health concerns, the work is not over. Maintaining good emotional health is a long-term project. Keep up with whatever therapy or group meetings help you. Continue practicing coping techniques. Life will always have ups and downs, but learning to face them sober is a skill that gets stronger with time.

It also helps to review your progress every few months. Ask yourself: How am I feeling overall? Have I noticed any old habits creeping back? Do I need a tune-up session with a counselor? Being proactive prevents a slip from turning into a full relapse, especially if old mental health patterns try to return.

7.17 Conclusion of Chapter 7

Mental health problems go hand-in-hand with alcohol use for many women. Anxiety, depression, and low self-esteem are common threads that keep a person trapped. Quitting can free up the brain and body to heal, but it also reveals emotions that might have been hidden by drinking. Seeking professional support, learning new coping skills, and connecting with others can lay the groundwork for true emotional well-being. No matter how bad things may seem, it is possible to reclaim a sense of balance and peace. The path might feel bumpy at first, but with the right tools and support, you can find steadier ground for both your mind and body.

Chapter 8: Breaking Old Patterns

8.1 Introduction: The Power of Habit

Everyone has habits, some good and some bad. Alcohol use can be one of those habits that become deeply ingrained over time. You might find yourself pouring a drink without even thinking, or automatically reaching for a glass when you feel stressed. These patterns can feel unshakable because they build mental ruts that are hard to climb out of. Yet, breaking old patterns is entirely possible. In this chapter, we explore how habits form, why they stick around, and practical methods to replace them with healthier actions.

8.2 How Habits Form in the Brain

The brain loves routines. They save energy and time. When you do something repeatedly—like grabbing a drink at the end of the day—your brain links that action with whatever reward it thinks it gets (such as relaxation or numbness). Over time, the neural pathways get stronger. This is why it is so hard to resist that end-of-day drink if it has become your routine.

Think of a habit as having three parts: a cue (something that triggers the habit), a routine (the action you take), and a reward (the payoff you feel). For drinking, the cue might be getting home from work or feeling angry. The routine is pouring a drink. The reward is the temporary relief or buzz. Breaking old patterns means interrupting this cycle. You can either change the routine or find a new way to get a similar reward.

8.3 Spotting Automatic Behaviors

One key step is spotting the automatic moments. These are the times when you act without thinking. For example, you might notice that the minute you walk into your kitchen, you head to the fridge for a beer. Or whenever you scroll through social media in the evening, you also sip a glass of wine. The more you pay attention, the more you see these actions are practically on autopilot.

It helps to keep a small journal or note on your phone. Jot down the time, place, and what you were feeling when you had the urge to drink. Doing this for a few weeks can reveal clear patterns. Maybe you see that 7 p.m. is always your breaking point, or that arguments with a spouse trigger a strong craving. Armed with this knowledge, you can plan changes.

8.4 Replacing the Habit with Something New

Most experts agree that to truly break an old habit, you should replace it rather than just remove it. The mind is used to the reward, so it wants something in place of that old action. For instance, if your habit is to watch TV with a glass of wine, try having a mug of herbal tea or seltzer water instead. It might not feel as rewarding at first, but over time, your brain can adjust. You could also fill that time with a pleasant distraction, like knitting or a light puzzle, so your hands are busy.

The idea is to keep the cue but change the routine. If the cue is finishing dinner, and you always reach for a drink, you could replace it with taking a short walk or playing a word game on your phone. The goal is to find something that offers a small reward (relaxation, fun, or a sense of achievement) without the damaging effects of alcohol.

8.5 Managing Cravings

Cravings are powerful urges that can seem impossible to resist. They often appear when your brain thinks it is missing out on the old habit. The trick is to view cravings like waves: they rise, peak, and then fall. If you hold on and find a distraction, the urge often passes in about 20 minutes. Some methods to manage cravings:

- **Drink a glass of water**: This gives you a moment to pause and might help lessen the craving.
- **Chew gum or suck on a mint**: These small actions can occupy your mouth and mind for a while.
- **Call or text someone**: Talking to a friend can shift your thoughts away from the craving.
- **Do a quick task**: Wash dishes, fold laundry, or walk up and down the stairs. Physical activity can disrupt the craving loop.

Over time, each time you resist a craving, you weaken its hold. You teach your brain that you do not need alcohol to satisfy that urge.

8.6 Changing Your Environment

Sometimes, the environment itself can lock you into old patterns. If you keep alcohol in the house, it is much easier to slip. If you always go to the same bar with friends, you will be more tempted. Changing your environment can break the habit loop. This might mean removing all alcohol from your home or rearranging the kitchen so there is no special "drink area." It could mean choosing a new route home from work so you do not pass by your usual liquor store.

It might also mean adjusting your social environment. If your circle of friends only meets up for drinks, consider suggesting different activities. If they are not open to that, you may need to limit your time with them until you feel stronger in your new habit. This can be tough, but it is a vital step for many women who want to break free from old patterns.

8.7 Gradual vs. Sudden Changes

Some women find success by cutting alcohol completely at once. Others prefer a gradual approach, reducing the amount or frequency over time. Both strategies can work, but it helps to know which style suits your personality and lifestyle. If you do better with clear rules, going "cold turkey" might help. If that feels too overwhelming, you could set smaller goals like "No drinks on weekdays" and slowly increase that boundary.

Either way, the key is to stay consistent. If you choose a gradual reduction but keep making excuses to drink more than planned, you might never reach your goal. If you go cold turkey but slip up, you might feel like a failure and quit trying. That is why having a plan in place for handling slip-ups is important. One mistake does not mean you have to abandon the whole effort.

8.8 The Problem of "Just One Drink"

"Just one drink" can be a tricky phrase. Some women think they can handle a single glass and stop. Sometimes, that works. But for many, "just one" opens the door to more. Once alcohol is in your system, your determination can weaken. You might say, "Well, I had one, so another won't hurt." Then it becomes three or four.

If you know that you struggle with stopping once you start, it might be safest to skip that first drink entirely. Even social occasions do not have to be a time for "just one." You can always choose a non-alcoholic beverage and still enjoy chatting or dancing. Over time, you may realize that the excitement you thought came from a drink is actually within you, not in the glass.

8.9 Setting Clear Goals

A good way to break old patterns is to set clear goals. Vague aims like "I want to drink less" are hard to follow. Instead, be specific: "I will not drink any alcohol for the next 30 days," or "I will not keep any alcohol in the house." These defined goals give you something firm to measure. You can mark progress on a calendar or app.

When setting goals, also think about what you want from this change. Is it better health, more money, or improved relationships? Write down these motivations. Looking at them can remind you why you started when you feel tempted to slip back into old habits.

8.10 Rewards for Success

Breaking old patterns can be challenging. Setting small rewards for milestones can boost your motivation. For example, if you go a whole week without a drink, treat yourself to something you enjoy—a new book, a spa day at home, or a nice meal. The reward should not involve alcohol, of course. The idea is to let your brain associate quitting with positive outcomes.

Some women worry that rewards are childish, but they can be quite helpful. Even giving yourself a gold star on a chart can spark a little bit of joy. Over time, your biggest reward will be feeling better, looking healthier, and having more control over your life. But these small treats along the way can keep you on track while you wait for those bigger changes to unfold.

8.11 Accountability Partners

Having someone to check in with can help you stay committed. This could be a friend, a family member, or an online support buddy who shares similar goals. Set up a regular time to talk or message. Share both your successes and struggles. Knowing someone else is aware of your goal can add a layer of motivation. It is no longer a secret that you can hide from.

You can also join support communities or groups where people discuss their progress in breaking old habits. Hearing others' stories can remind you that you are not alone. It also allows you to learn from their mistakes and triumphs. Accountability is about mutual support, so be there for your partner as well, if possible.

8.12 Dealing with Emotional Ups and Downs

As you break old patterns, emotions may jump around. You might feel proud one day and frustrated the next. These ups and downs are normal because you are changing how your brain responds to daily life. Alcohol used to mask or soften certain feelings, so you might be experiencing them in full force now.

During low moments, remind yourself that these feelings pass. If sadness or anger is too strong to handle alone, consider talking to a counselor or therapist. Friends can also be a sounding board. Recognize that feeling emotions fully is a part of living without alcohol. Over time, you will learn healthier ways to process them.

8.13 Learning from Slip-Ups

It is common to have a slip-up on the road to breaking old patterns. You might go weeks without a drink and then, during a stressful day, have one. While it feels discouraging, slip-ups can be a chance to learn. Ask yourself what led to that moment. Was it a sudden burst of stress? Did you skip your usual coping methods?

By examining the slip-up, you can spot holes in your plan. Maybe you need a stronger back-up strategy for dealing with stress at work. Or maybe you need to leave social events earlier. Whatever it is, a slip-up does not erase all your progress. Treat it like a lesson. Strengthen your approach and keep going.

8.14 Long-Term Behavior Change

Breaking old patterns is not a one-time event. It is an ongoing process. In the first few weeks, you might rely on constant reminders and strategies. After a few months, new routines start to feel more natural. But remain attentive. Some women get overconfident and think they can handle a few drinks because they have changed so much. That can be risky if it leads to falling back into old ways.

Over the long term, you might find new interests or activities that replace the time and energy you used to devote to drinking. You might pick up a hobby, learn a language, or volunteer in your community. These new passions give you a sense of purpose that makes the idea of drinking less appealing.

8.15 The Role of Positive Self-Talk

Self-talk refers to the thoughts you direct at yourself. Negative self-talk might sound like, "I'm never going to break this pattern," or "I'm weak for giving in to cravings." Positive self-talk, on the other hand, encourages and builds you up. It might say, "I handled that stress without alcohol—good job," or "I slipped once, but I'm back on track, and that's what matters."

Changing your self-talk can be tricky at first because negative thoughts might pop up automatically. But you can replace them with more balanced ones. For instance, if you catch yourself thinking, "I'll never get this right," you can reframe it: "Change is hard, but I'm making progress every day." This shift can reduce discouragement and help keep you focused on your goal.

8.16 Creating a Personal Action Plan

To tie it all together, create a personal action plan for breaking old patterns. It might look like this:

1. **Identify cues**: List when and where you usually feel the urge to drink.
2. **Replace routines**: Decide what action you will take instead. (Tea, walk, hobby, phone call, etc.)
3. **Plan for cravings**: Keep items like gum or mints handy. Have a go-to activity ready.
4. **Adjust environment**: Remove or hide alcohol, choose different social settings, or limit contact with people who pressure you.
5. **Set goals and rewards**: Be clear on what you want to achieve, and plan small rewards for meeting milestones.
6. **Use accountability**: Pick a person or group to report to on a regular basis.
7. **Review progress**: Check in weekly or monthly to see what is working and what needs adjusting.

Having everything written down makes it real. You can refer back to the plan when you feel unsure. This also helps you see how far you have come.

8.17 Conclusion of Chapter 8

Breaking old patterns of drinking is about more than just willpower. It is about understanding how habits form, learning to spot the cues, and replacing the routine with something healthier. It takes time, patience, and self-kindness. By monitoring cravings, adjusting your environment, and setting clear goals, you can chip away at even the most ingrained habits. Remember, a slip-up or bad day does not undo your entire effort. Each small step forward can build on the last, leading to a life where alcohol no longer controls your choices or your mood.

Chapter 9: New Approaches to Handling Stress

9.1 Introduction: Why Stress Matters

Stress is an everyday part of life. It can come from work, family duties, money worries, or even small things like traffic jams. While some stress can motivate us to handle challenges, too much stress can harm the mind and body. Women who drink often list stress as one of their top reasons for reaching for a glass. They say it helps them forget problems or calm down. However, alcohol does not truly fix stress. It covers it up for a moment and often brings more issues later, such as health troubles or family conflicts.

In this chapter, we look at better ways to handle stress. These approaches are practical and can fit into everyday life. They do not require special tools or big budgets. The aim is to show that you can face problems without needing a drink. Over time, your mind will learn new responses, and stress will not feel as crushing.

9.2 Understanding How Stress Builds Up

It helps to know what stress does to the body. When we sense a threat or challenge, the brain releases hormones that put us in a "fight or flight" state. These hormones raise our heart rate and make us more alert. In the past, this was useful when humans needed to run from wild animals. Today, our threats might be arguments at home, work deadlines, or financial pressure. The body does not see the difference. It reacts the same way.

When stress keeps happening, the body stays on high alert. This can lead to headaches, tension, poor sleep, or anger. If you do not find healthy ways to handle it, you might turn to quick fixes like alcohol. But that only delays facing the real issues. Learning new methods can break this cycle, giving you the power to respond better.

9.3 Breathing Exercises and Quick Relaxation

Many people overlook the value of a simple deep breath. When you feel stress climbing, a few slow inhales and exhales can lower your heart rate and calm the mind. One method is called "4-4-4-4." You inhale for four counts, hold for four, exhale for four, and pause for four before inhaling again. Repeat several times. It might feel silly at first, but it can relax the body quickly.

Another idea is to place a hand on your stomach while you breathe. Aim to make your belly expand on each inhale. This type of breathing sends a signal to your brain that you are safe. Over time, your body starts to leave the "fight or flight" mode. You might also try closing your eyes and picturing a peaceful place, like a calm lake or a quiet forest. This gives your mind something soothing to focus on instead of stressful thoughts.

9.4 Moving the Body to Ease Tension

Physical movement is one of the best ways to let go of stress. It does not have to be a heavy workout. Simple activities like walking, stretching, or dancing around the house can help. When you move, your body uses up stress hormones and releases chemicals that make you feel better. This is why people often describe feeling happier or calmer after a short walk.

If you want something structured, you can try a low-impact exercise routine. There are many free videos online that guide you through gentle workouts. Some people also find relief in simple routines that involve slow movements and calm breathing. The goal is not to become an athlete but to release built-up tension. Over time, regular movement can make your body stronger and help you cope with daily worries more effectively.

9.5 Helpful Routines for the Morning

How you start the day can set the tone for everything that follows. If you jump out of bed late, skip breakfast, and rush off to work, you might feel hurried and frazzled. This stress can build up and make you want a drink by evening. Instead, try waking up a bit earlier. You could spend a few minutes doing a calm activity—like reading a few pages of a simple book or sipping a warm drink while looking out a window. You can also take a moment to write down a quick plan for the day, noting the top tasks you want to handle.

Some women find it useful to do a few stretches right after they get out of bed. This wakes up the muscles gently. Others like to listen to soft music or a relaxing audio program while they get dressed. The point is to give your mind and body a little calm time before jumping into your responsibilities. This small change can lower your stress load for the rest of the day.

9.6 Time Management as Stress Control

One big source of stress is feeling that there is not enough time. Many women juggle work, family, household chores, and personal tasks. They end the day exhausted and look for an escape, which can lead to drinking. Good time management can relieve some of this pressure. Start by making a list of everything you need to do. Then, prioritize tasks. Which are urgent? Which can wait? Which can be done in smaller steps?

You might also need to say no to extra demands. If someone asks you to take on more work, and you already feel overloaded, it is okay to decline. Setting boundaries is not selfish; it is necessary for your well-being. By organizing your time, you reduce chaos and make space for short breaks. This can prevent the kind of stress buildup that pushes you to seek a quick fix.

9.7 Mental Breaks and Mindful Moments

During the day, it is easy to let stress creep in. You might get an email that frustrates you or an unexpected chore pops up. Taking mental breaks helps keep stress from piling too high. A mental break can be as short as 30 seconds, where you close your eyes, breathe deeply, and let your mind settle. Some women like to step outside for a moment, look at the sky, or feel the breeze.

"Mindful moments" are similar but can happen during everyday activities. For instance, if you are washing dishes, pay attention to the water's temperature and the soap's smell. Let yourself be there in the moment, instead of worrying about other tasks. It may seem basic, but focusing on a single task like this quiets the racing mind. Over time, practicing this can reduce overall stress because you train yourself to stay in the present.

9.8 Relaxing Activities and Hobbies

Many people who quit drinking discover they have more free time. What you do with that time can affect your stress levels. Choosing relaxing or enjoyable hobbies can be a great outlet. Maybe you like drawing, reading mystery novels, or tending to indoor plants. Others might enjoy cooking new recipes or doing simple crafts.

If you do not have a clear hobby, think about what interests you. Is there something you used to enjoy as a kid? Sometimes, coloring books for adults can help calm the mind. If you are more active, you might try bike rides or a slow jog. The point is to do something that is not tied to alcohol and helps your brain focus on a pleasant task. This can lower stress and give you something to look forward to each day.

9.9 Talking it Out with Someone Trustworthy

Holding in worries can make stress worse. Sharing your thoughts with a friend, family member, or counselor can relieve some of the burden. You do not need to have a big, formal talk. Sometimes just calling a friend to say, "I'm having a hard day" can be enough to release tension. If you do not feel comfortable talking to someone you know, consider an online support group where you can talk anonymously.

Therapy or counseling can also help if stress feels unmanageable. A professional can guide you in spotting patterns and teach you practical tools to use when you feel overwhelmed. This might include problem-solving strategies or simple mental tasks to calm down. Talking about your struggles is not a sign of weakness; it shows you are taking steps to handle stress in a healthy way.

9.10 Writing as a Release

Some women find it hard to talk about their worries but easier to write them down. You can keep a small journal or even use a notebook app on your phone. When you feel stressed, jot down what is bothering you. It does not have to be perfect or well organized. The act of putting thoughts into words often reduces their power. After writing, you might notice you feel calmer or have a clearer idea of what to do next.

You can use writing as a daily habit. Each evening, spend five minutes writing about what went right that day, what felt hard, and how you handled it. This helps you see patterns in your stress. Maybe you notice that late afternoon is always tough, or that certain people trigger frustration. By noticing these patterns, you can plan better responses.

9.11 Learning to Say "No"

Many women feel guilty when they say no. They might worry about disappointing others or appear lazy. But taking on too many commitments can wear you down. If you are always saying yes, you might find your schedule is so packed that you have no time to rest. This constant state of rush can drive you to seek relief in a drink.

Practice saying no in a polite but firm way. For instance, "I'm sorry, I won't be able to handle that right now." Or, "I appreciate the offer, but I have too much on my plate." You do not need to give a detailed explanation. Most reasonable people will respect your honesty. By setting these limits, you free up mental space and cut back on stressful overload.

9.12 Tending to Physical Health

Physical health and stress are closely linked. When you eat better, stay hydrated, and get enough sleep, your body can handle stress more easily. If your body is run down, small problems will feel bigger. Many women who drink have poor sleep patterns. Quitting alcohol can help restore healthy rest. Combine that with a balanced diet, and you may see a drop in your stress levels.

Think about simple dietary changes. Swap out sugary snacks for fruits or nuts. Drink enough water throughout the day. These changes might seem small, but they can make a big difference in how you feel. When your body is strong, it can cope better with life's demands. A run-down body might respond to stress with headaches, muscle tension, or mood swings, which again can push you to seek escape in alcohol.

9.13 Breaking the Cycle of Self-Criticism

Stress can also come from within. Some women put themselves down with harsh self-talk, like "I'm not good enough" or "I always mess up." This inner criticism can add a layer of stress to everything you do. The next time you catch a negative thought, pause and replace it with a balanced statement. For instance, if you think, "I'm failing at work," you can tell yourself, "I had a tough day, but I handled it as best as I could, and I can do better tomorrow."

Over time, this gentler self-talk eases internal tension. You stop being your own worst critic and start becoming your own supporter. This does not mean ignoring mistakes. It means acknowledging them without adding layers of shame. Healthy self-talk can turn stress into a manageable problem rather than a crisis that drives you toward a drink.

9.14 Social Connections and Support

Having supportive people around can cut stress levels. Good friends, kind neighbors, or understanding coworkers can all provide a sense of belonging. When you face a stressful event, you can lean on them for help or just to vent. If you do not have a strong social network, it might be time to build one. You can join community groups or clubs that match your interests. You could volunteer somewhere, meeting people who share your values.

Online communities can also play a role. There are many forums where women share their efforts in quitting drinking and handling stress. Reading their stories or joining conversations can reduce feelings of isolation. It also gives you new insights and ideas for handling everyday tension.

9.15 Calm Evenings and Better Wind-Down Routines

Many women find the evening is when their stress peaks. After a long day, they feel drained and want instant relief. This can lead to the nightly glass (or bottle) of wine. A better approach is to set up a wind-down routine that does not involve alcohol. Maybe you take a warm shower, change into comfortable clothes, and spend a few minutes reading. Some people find playing soft music while tidying up the house helps them transition to bedtime.

Dim the lights, avoid looking at bright screens too close to bed, and think of a calming activity. This signals the brain that it is time to slow down. If you have a partner or family members, you can ask them to join you in a calm evening hour—no loud TV, no arguments, and no last-minute chores. This can reduce your overall stress and help you get better quality sleep.

9.16 Trying Out Small Changes First

If changing everything at once feels overwhelming, pick one or two ideas from this chapter to start with. Maybe begin with five-minute breathing breaks or decide to say no to one extra commitment this week. Even small steps can lower your stress a bit, which reduces the urge to drink. As you see these small successes, you can add more changes.

It is also okay if certain methods do not work for you. Everyone is different. You might find that writing helps you more than breathing exercises, or that talking to a friend calms you better than going for a walk. The key is to keep trying different approaches until you discover what feels right and brings real relief.

9.17 Conclusion of Chapter 9

Stress is a major reason many women reach for alcohol. By learning new approaches, you can face stress head-on rather than masking it with a drink. Methods like breathing exercises, simple movement, mindful routines, and positive self-talk can all lessen the load. You do not have to become a stress-free person overnight. The goal is to find small actions that make a real difference. Over time, these healthy habits can replace the old pattern of turning to alcohol. Then, stress becomes something you manage, not something that rules your life.

Chapter 10: Practical Ways to Avoid Triggers

10.1 Introduction: Recognizing the Power of Triggers

A trigger is anything—an event, a place, a feeling—that prompts the urge to drink. For some women, it might be passing by a liquor store. For others, it might be feeling lonely or hearing a certain song that reminds them of past drinking days. Triggers are powerful because they can override your resolve in seconds. If you do not learn how to handle them, they can pull you back to old habits again and again.

This chapter offers concrete methods to avoid triggers or manage them better if you cannot avoid them altogether. The goal is not to live in constant fear but to plan ahead. When you know your triggers, you can create strategies to stay on track. Over time, triggers lose some of their power, and you build confidence in your ability to choose not to drink.

10.2 Finding Your Personal Triggers

The first step is to identify what sets off your cravings. Triggers fall into a few main categories:

1. **Places**: Bars, certain restaurants, or even your own living room if that is where you used to drink.
2. **People**: Friends who encourage you to drink, family members who cause you stress, or a partner who drinks in front of you.
3. **Emotions**: Anger, sadness, boredom, or anxiety.
4. **Times of day**: Maybe the craving hits after dinner or before bedtime.
5. **Events or Celebrations**: Holidays, birthdays, or social gatherings can trigger old patterns.

Make a list of these triggers. Write them down as specifically as possible. For example, instead of "sadness," write "feeling sad on Sunday evenings because the weekend is ending." The more detail you include, the clearer your plan can be.

10.3 Physical Avoidance Tactics

One straightforward way to reduce triggers is to change your physical environment. If you know a certain bar on your way home always lures you in, pick a different route. If you often drank in your kitchen, consider rearranging it. Remove any alcohol-related glasses or decorations that spark the urge. If you are used to sitting in a particular chair with a drink, move the chair or replace it.

You can also remove alcohol from your home. If you live with others who still drink, ask them to keep it in a less visible spot or in a locked cupboard. Out of sight often helps lessen the urge. The fewer visual reminders around, the less likely you are to slip into an automatic habit. These changes might feel odd at first, but they can make a big difference, especially in the early stages of quitting.

10.4 Handling Social Circles

People can be a strong trigger. Maybe you have friends who bond over weekly wine nights, or relatives who always hand you a drink at family gatherings. If being around these folks makes it hard to resist drinking, you might need to set limits. This does not mean cutting them off entirely (unless they are truly harmful influences). But you can choose how and when to see them.

For instance, if a friend always wants to meet at a bar, you can suggest meeting at a coffee shop or taking a walk in the park. If they insist on drinking, you can either attend briefly or skip the event until you feel stronger in your resolve. Some women find that certain friendships revolve only around alcohol. This can be a harsh truth to face, but letting go of such friendships can be vital if you want to stay sober.

10.5 Emotional Triggers: Creating a Coping Toolbox

Emotions like sadness, stress, or loneliness can drive the urge to drink. If you know a certain feeling is a trigger, create a "coping toolbox." This is a set of go-to methods or items that help you handle the emotion in a healthier way. For example, if loneliness strikes, you might pull out your phone and call a supportive friend or join an online chat group. If stress is the culprit, you could use the breathing exercises mentioned in Chapter 9.

You might also include small items in your toolbox, like a stress ball, a doodle pad, or a list of soothing music you can play. The idea is to have options ready so you do not scramble at the last minute. Keeping a list of phone numbers for hotlines or local support groups is another smart addition. Then, when the emotion hits, you have a plan that does not involve running to a drink.

10.6 Time-Based Triggers

Many women find that certain times of day are more tempting. It could be right after work, late at night, or when the kids go to bed. If you know this about yourself, schedule something else during that time. For instance, if you feel the urge right after you get home, plan a 15-minute walk before entering your house. Or prepare a light, relaxing task for yourself, like listening to a short audio program.

You can also shift your dinner time or bedtime routines to break the old pattern. If you used to have a glass of wine after dinner, try taking a bath or reading a chapter of a book right after your meal. Making small changes to your schedule can disrupt the automatic habit of drinking at a certain hour.

10.7 Event Triggers and Social Gatherings

Parties, holidays, and special gatherings can be major triggers. Everyone might be toasting with champagne, or friends might show up with bottles of wine. To handle these events, plan well in advance. Let the host know you will not be drinking. Offer to bring your own non-alcoholic beverages. This way, you are not stuck sipping water while everyone else has something fancy.

If you feel pressured to participate in a toast, you can raise a glass of sparkling water or juice. Often, people do not notice or care as much as you might fear. If anyone asks, you can simply say, "I'm not drinking these days," without giving a full explanation. If the event becomes overwhelming, it is also okay to leave early. Having an exit plan (like driving yourself or arranging a ride) can reduce anxiety about being trapped in a place where triggers abound.

10.8 Urge Surfing: Learning to Ride Out Cravings

"Urge surfing" is a method where you notice the craving, accept that it is happening, and wait for it to peak and fall without acting on it. Think of a craving as a wave in the ocean. It starts small, builds up, and eventually breaks. If you do not feed the craving by drinking, it will pass. You do not push the wave away or deny it; you just observe it.

To do this, find a quiet space when a craving hits. Close your eyes, if possible, and focus on what the urge feels like. Maybe your mouth waters, or you feel tension in your chest. Notice these sensations without trying to change them. Breathe slowly. Remind yourself that urges come and go. Many people find that after a few minutes, the craving weakens on its own. This approach can build mental strength and help you realize that cravings are temporary signals, not unstoppable forces.

10.9 Involving Allies

It is easier to avoid triggers when you have people on your side. This might include a spouse or a close friend who respects your decision to quit. Ask them to help you avoid tricky situations. For instance, if you are going to a party together, they can offer to leave with you if the environment becomes too tempting. They can also help steer conversations away from drinking.

If you are living with someone who still drinks, talk openly about your concerns. Maybe they can agree not to drink around you for a while. Or they can store their drinks in a separate area. Knowing that a loved one is willing to support you can reduce the stress of dealing with triggers alone. You might also find local support groups or online groups where you can post about upcoming events and get advice from others who have been in the same spot.

10.10 Creating New Routines in Old Spaces

Sometimes, triggers are not just about the presence of alcohol, but about the memory of drinking in certain places. Maybe you always drank on your porch at sunset or in your living room while watching TV. To break that link, create a new routine in that same space. For instance, if you used to sit on the porch with a drink, bring out a crossword puzzle or a coloring book instead. Listen to a podcast or chat with a friend on the phone. Slowly, your mind will start to link that space with other activities.

You can also change how the space looks. Move the furniture, add some plants, or hang a new picture on the wall. These small changes can reset the mental cues that used to say, "Time to drink." Over time, your brain adjusts to the new use of that space, and the craving becomes less intense.

10.11 Handling Unexpected Triggers

Not all triggers are predictable. You might run into an old friend who invites you for a drink, or you see an emotional scene on TV that stirs up tough memories. The best defense is having a general plan for sudden temptations. This could include a statement you say to yourself, such as, "I do not drink anymore, even if I feel tempted right now." Or you might quickly send a message to a supportive friend, saying, "I need help. I just got triggered."

Carrying a small item in your pocket or purse can also help. Some people keep a reminder card with reasons they quit drinking. Others keep a short note that says, "Your future matters more than this craving." This quick reference can ground you in a moment of surprise. By having a ready response, you will not be caught off guard, and you can hold steady until the urge passes.

10.12 Changing How You Think About Alcohol

A deep part of managing triggers is changing your mindset. If you secretly believe alcohol is the best way to relax or have fun, triggers will always hold a strong pull. But if you start seeing alcohol as a problem that harmed your life, the mental appeal weakens. You can remind yourself of the negative effects it had: lost money, strained relationships, or health worries. Each time a trigger appears, bring those memories to the forefront.

You might also list the positives of staying sober: clearer thoughts, better health, happier family members, and more free time. Seeing alcohol as something you no longer want in your life can lessen the impact of triggers. Over time, the mental shift can be so strong that you feel little to no attraction when confronted with old cues.

10.13 Rewards for Overcoming Triggers

Just like in the previous chapter about breaking old patterns, rewards can help you stay motivated. Each time you handle a trigger successfully, give yourself a small treat. It does not need to be big or cost a lot. It might be a simple activity you enjoy—like watching a short comedy clip, reading an extra chapter of a book, or having a favorite snack. This tells your brain that resisting triggers leads to positive outcomes.

You can also keep track of how many triggers you faced in a week and how many times you resisted. Seeing the number of "wins" can boost your confidence. You might share these victories in a support group or with a friend who cheers you on. Feeling proud of your ability to stay sober in the face of triggers is a powerful reward on its own.

10.14 Learning from Slip-Ups

Avoiding triggers is a skill, and you might not be perfect at it right away. If you slip and have a drink, do not view it as a permanent failure. Instead, ask what happened. Which trigger caught you off guard? Did you have a plan, and did you follow it? Was there something else you could have done? This self-check helps you refine your trigger strategy.

You might realize you need to avoid certain people or places for a longer time until you feel more stable. Or you might see that you need more robust emotional support. Use slip-ups as a learning tool, not a reason to give up. Over time, these lessons will help you build a rock-solid approach to triggers.

10.15 Consistency Over the Long Haul

When you first quit, triggers can feel very strong. But as the weeks and months pass, the urge often fades. Consistency is key. Keep up with the methods that work. If you find that rearranging your living room helped, stick with it. If you discover that calling a friend is the best way to handle emotional triggers, do it every time. The more you use these tools, the more natural they become.

Eventually, you might feel comfortable in situations that used to be dangerous. However, do not let your guard down completely. Some women find that a big life event—like a loss or a major change—can reignite triggers. Stay aware of your patterns, and keep your strategies fresh in your mind. This awareness does not mean living in fear. It just means you respect the power of triggers enough to be prepared.

10.16 Looking Forward: Building a Life Beyond Triggers

The ultimate goal is to reach a point where triggers do not rule your decisions. You might still notice them, but you can choose how to respond. This opens the door to a more fulfilling life. You can make plans without thinking, "Will I drink?" or "How do I avoid drinking?" You reclaim your time and energy for things that matter to you: hobbies, family, career goals, or personal growth.

This does not happen overnight, but every time you resist a trigger, you take another step in that direction. The pride and self-trust that come from beating triggers build up. One day, you may realize that what used to tempt you now feels unimportant. That is the sign of real progress and freedom.

10.17 Conclusion of Chapter 10

Triggers are a normal part of the process when quitting alcohol. They can pop up in the form of people, places, emotions, or even old memories. Learning to avoid or handle them is a skill that can grow with practice. By identifying your triggers, adjusting your surroundings, involving supportive people, and practicing urge surfing, you can stand firm against cravings. Over time, triggers lose their hold, and you gain confidence in living without alcohol.

These practical tactics, combined with the stress-handling ideas from Chapter 9, lay a strong foundation for long-term success. You do not have to hide away from the world. You just need a plan, some support, and a fresh viewpoint on what alcohol represents in your life. Keep refining your methods, reward yourself for each win, and use any slip-up as a lesson. Gradually, you will see that you can face triggers with calm and stay true to your goal of living free from alcohol.

Chapter 11: Setting Up a Strong Support System

11.1 Introduction: Why Support Matters

Quitting alcohol can feel like a big task. You might be dealing with cravings, social pressures, and deep habits you have formed over the years. One factor that can help you in a major way is having a strong support system. This means having people, groups, or services that stand by you and make the path easier to manage. You do not have to do everything on your own. A network of allies can boost your resolve when your willpower runs low.

In this chapter, we will look at different types of support—ranging from close friends and family to professional services and online communities. We will talk about how to find them, how to ask for help, and how to maintain healthy, respectful boundaries. The aim is to equip you with concrete steps so you know whom to turn to and what to do when you feel unsteady.

11.2 Recognizing the Need for Help

Many women think they must handle problems alone. They might feel that asking for assistance is a sign of weakness or that nobody else cares about what they are going through. These thoughts can keep you isolated, making it easier to slip back into old drinking habits when stress or loneliness hits.

Recognizing you need help is the first step. This can look like noticing you often feel tempted to drink when upset, or you have tried to quit multiple times without success. It can also mean you do not have anyone to talk to about cravings or emotional concerns. At this point, telling yourself "I cannot do this all alone" is a healthy step toward building a support system.

11.3 Types of Support Systems

Support can come in many forms. Each has its own strengths, and you may find you need more than one kind:

1. **Close Friends and Family**: These are people who know you well and have a personal bond with you. They can offer encouragement, check up on you, and cheer on your progress.
2. **Support Groups**: These can be face-to-face meetings or online forums where individuals share their experiences. People here understand your struggles because they have faced similar challenges.
3. **Professional Help**: This includes therapists, counselors, medical experts, and social workers who can guide you with structured methods and knowledge about addiction and mental health.
4. **Faith or Community Organizations**: Some people find help through local community centers, religious groups, or charitable groups that focus on personal improvement.
5. **Sober Companions or Mentors**: In some places, there are programs that match you with someone who is further along in quitting. They can give tips and check in with you regularly.

You do not have to choose just one source of help. Combining two or three types can give you a stronger safety net. If one source is busy or not responding, another might be available, so you never feel totally alone.

11.4 Talking to Family and Friends

If your family members or closest friends are understanding, they can be a huge help. However, you will need to communicate clearly about your decision to quit drinking. Many people assume their loved ones know what is happening, but that is often not the case. Sit down with them if you can and explain why you are stopping. Let them know the kind of support you want. This could be:

- **Practical Support**: Not offering you drinks at gatherings, or not drinking around you for a while.
- **Emotional Support**: Listening when you need to talk, checking in with you if they sense you are stressed.
- **Accountability**: Asking you regularly about your progress, or stepping in if they notice signs you might relapse.

Some might be excited to help, while others may not grasp the seriousness. They might say, "Oh, you can have just one drink." If they do not understand, stay calm and restate your decision. It might take time for them to see you are serious. If a loved one drinks heavily themselves, you may have to set extra limits to protect your sobriety.

11.5 Finding or Forming a Support Group

For many women, a support group is a key part of staying sober. In these settings, you meet people who share their stories about quitting or cutting back. Hearing how someone else handled tough cravings can give you fresh ideas. Plus, a group provides a place to speak openly about struggles without judgment.

Some well-known groups meet in person. Others function online, which is helpful if you live far from a meeting location or prefer private discussions. Online forums let you chat anytime, day or night. This can be crucial if a craving strikes late in the evening and you do not have anyone else to call.

If you cannot find a group in your area, think about starting one. You might reach out to local community centers, libraries, or churches to see if they have space for a small weekly meeting. Even if you gather only a few people at first, it can grow over time. The main idea is to create a safe environment where everyone can be honest and supportive.

11.6 Professional Services: Therapists and Counselors

Sometimes, a woman needs more than casual support. This is where professional help comes in. A therapist or counselor trained in alcohol misuse can guide you in understanding why you drink, how to handle triggers, and how to build healthier coping skills. They offer a private space to discuss emotions you might not feel comfortable sharing with friends.

Therapy might involve talking about past traumas, relationships, or mental health issues like anxiety or sadness. This can be intense, but it often leads to deep change. A skilled therapist will not judge you. Instead, they will work with you on plans to avoid relapse and to build a better life. If you have medical concerns about withdrawal or mental health, seeing a professional can be crucial. In some cases, they might suggest medication or specialized treatment programs.

11.7 Online Communities and Social Media Support

The internet has made it easier to find groups worldwide. Platforms exist where members share daily updates, exchange tips, and send encouragement. Some are general "quit drinking" groups. Others focus on women's needs specifically, giving a space to talk about body image, child care, or relationship dynamics that might be linked to drinking.

The advantage of online communities is availability. You can post at midnight if a craving hits. You can read through old threads where people faced similar situations. This sense of being heard can reduce feelings of isolation. However, be careful with the credibility of advice online. Not everyone is a licensed professional. Also, maintain your privacy. Use a nickname or partial name if you prefer, so you can speak openly without concern for anyone recognizing you.

11.8 Accountability Partners

An accountability partner is someone you choose to update regularly. This could be a friend, a fellow group member, or a trained mentor. You agree on how often you will check in—maybe daily messages or a phone call every few days. During these check-ins, you share your recent wins, struggles, or upcoming challenges. The partner does the same if it is a mutual arrangement.

This setup works well for many women because it adds a layer of commitment. Knowing that someone will ask, "Did you stay sober today?" can make you pause before you pick up a drink. It also means you have someone to call if you are feeling shaky. You do not have to wonder whom to reach out to. Your accountability partner is expecting to hear from you.

11.9 Handling Negative or Unsupportive People

Not everyone will be on your side. You might have friends who tease you for quitting, or family members who do not believe alcohol is really a problem. Perhaps they feel threatened by your choice because it makes them examine their own drinking. Negative folks might make remarks such as, "You are overreacting," or "You used to be more fun."

It can be hurtful, especially if these are people you care about. You have a few choices. If possible, you can limit the time you spend with them until you feel stronger in your sobriety. If that is not possible, prepare short responses. For example, if someone says, "Just have one drink," you might say, "No, thanks, that is not an option for me." Then change the topic or walk away. You have the right to protect your well-being.

11.10 Setting Boundaries for Lasting Support

Boundaries are rules or limits you set for how others treat you and how you spend your time. They keep your support system healthy. For instance, you might tell a friend you cannot stay out late at bars with her anymore because it tempts you to drink. Or you might ask family members not to bring alcohol into your home.

At first, some people may not understand why you need these boundaries. They might take it personally. However, if they truly care about you, they will adapt. Boundaries do more than protect you from negative influence. They also encourage healthier interactions in all areas of life. Over time, these limits help you maintain your progress and keep harmful habits at bay.

11.11 Using Tech Tools to Stay Connected

In today's world, there are many apps and digital tools that can aid your support system. You can find trackers that let you log each day sober. Some apps allow you to chat with other members who are also quitting. Others send motivational quotes or daily tips. If you already use a calendar app, you can set reminders to check in with your accountability partner or attend a meeting.

Tech tools are not a substitute for real human contact, but they can fill gaps when you need quick inspiration. For example, if you feel a craving coming on, you might open your sober tracker app and see a list of reasons you quit. Some apps even have built-in panic buttons. If you are at risk of relapse, you can press the button to connect with a volunteer or professional who can talk you through the moment.

11.12 When to Consider Structured Treatment Programs

For some women, casual support or a bit of therapy might not be enough. If you have tried multiple times to quit and keep falling back into heavy drinking, a structured program could help. This might include inpatient or outpatient rehab centers where professionals offer round-the-clock guidance. These programs often involve group sessions, one-on-one counseling, and classes on coping skills.

Structured programs can also address any medical issues tied to withdrawal. If you have been drinking for a long time, stopping suddenly can lead to symptoms like tremors, anxiety, or even seizures in extreme cases. Medical staff at a rehab center can monitor you. They might prescribe medication to ease this transition. While rehab can be costly, insurance sometimes covers part or all of it. There are also state-funded options for those who qualify financially. Do not let cost concerns stop you from exploring whether rehab might be the right fit.

11.13 Balancing Independence and Support

While having a support system is vital, it is also important to develop personal accountability. You do not want to rely on others so heavily that you cannot function alone. The best approach is a blend: you turn to people or services when you are in a tight spot, but you also learn to handle smaller challenges by yourself.

For example, if you face a mild craving on a normal day, you might do some breathing exercises or distract yourself with an activity. If the craving grows intense or you encounter a major crisis, then you call a friend or professional. Over time, you build confidence in your own coping skills. When you see that you can handle certain triggers without external help, you feel stronger. This sense of personal power can push you forward toward your bigger goals.

11.14 Adapting as You Grow

Your support system might change as you progress. Early on, you might need daily check-ins with a friend, weekly therapy, and online group chats. After several months, you might find you only need therapy once a month and check in with your accountability partner once a week. It all depends on your comfort level and how stable you feel in your new habits.

Also, if you move to a different city or your schedule changes (like starting a new job), you might need to find new sources of help. This is normal. The key is not to assume you no longer need support just because you have had success for a while. Stay attentive to your feelings. If you start having more cravings or see old habits creeping back, reach out before a slip becomes a full relapse.

11.15 Healthy Communication in Your Support Network

Clear communication keeps your support network strong. If a friend does something that makes you uneasy—like offering you a drink "as a joke"—tell them calmly how that affects you. Do not let resentment build up. Also, be willing to listen if someone in your support group points out concerning signs in you. They might notice you are missing meetings or avoiding topics. Take their observations seriously.

Disagreements can happen in any close relationship. If you argue with your accountability partner, try to resolve it in a way that keeps the partnership intact. Remember, you share a goal: maintaining sobriety. Approach conflicts with the mindset of problem-solving, not blame. This approach helps ensure your support system remains solid even when misunderstandings occur.

11.16 Support for Additional Challenges

Some women face extra challenges on top of quitting, such as raising children alone, dealing with an unsupportive partner, or managing a tight budget. In such cases, your support system might include resources like childcare help, financial counseling, or legal aid. Do not hesitate to seek specialized services if you are dealing with complex problems.

Community centers often have lists of local resources. Online searches can also turn up free or low-cost help in your area. Though it might feel like too many steps, tackling these challenges can lower your stress, which in turn lowers your risk of relapse. For instance, if you find affordable childcare, you might have time to attend a support meeting or therapy session. If you get debt advice, you can reduce money stress that might push you to drink.

11.17 Conclusion of Chapter 11

A strong support system is like a safety net. It catches you when you stumble and gives you a sense of security. Whether it is a best friend you text daily, a counselor you see each week, or a local group where you share experiences, these connections can make your efforts more successful. Quitting does not have to be a lonely act. Reaching out for help is smart and often necessary.

As you build your network, remember to keep boundaries clear. Seek out people who respect your choices, offer genuine help, and understand that quitting is a serious commitment. Over time, your support system will become a core part of your new, healthier life. You will learn who you can turn to for practical aid, who can give you honest advice, and who lifts you up emotionally when times get hard.

Having set up a support network, the next step is learning how to fill your free time in ways that strengthen your resolve. Chapter 12 will cover how to shift habits and find interests that keep you active, content, and away from the habit of drinking. From leisure pursuits to personal growth projects, you will see that life without alcohol can be richer than you ever imagined.

Chapter 12: Making Better Use of Free Time

12.1 Introduction: A New View of Free Hours

When drinking was a regular habit, it might have taken up a lot of your free time. Maybe you met friends at bars, drank at home in the evenings, or spent weekends recovering from hangovers. Once you quit, those hours can feel empty. Some women find themselves at a loss about what to do. They might feel restless, bored, or even lonely.

This chapter focuses on how to fill your free time in ways that leave you feeling satisfied and motivated. When you find wholesome activities you enjoy, your mind is occupied, and cravings are less likely. Plus, you can rediscover old interests or explore new ones you never tried before. Using your free time wisely can be a powerful tool in staying sober for the long run.

12.2 Understanding the Role of Free Time in Relapse

Free time is often a double-edged sword. On one hand, it is a chance to relax, explore hobbies, and spend time with loved ones. On the other hand, if you are used to drinking during those moments, you might feel tempted to slip back into old patterns. Idle hours can be the toughest to handle because the mind starts wandering. You might think, "A drink would make this more fun," or "I'm so bored, so why not have a glass?"

By planning ahead for how you will use your free time, you lower the risk of these thoughts taking over. Having activities lined up—whether physical or mental—gives you a sense of purpose. Instead of feeling empty, you can look forward to something you truly like or something that moves you toward personal goals.

12.3 Recalling Old Passions

Think back to your younger days. Were there activities you loved but gave up along the way? Maybe you used to write short stories, play a musical instrument, or paint pictures. Quitting drinking can open the door to reigniting those past passions. Picking them up again might feel awkward at first if you are out of practice, but it can also spark joy as you reconnect with something that once mattered to you.

If you have trouble remembering old passions, try flipping through pictures or talking to old friends. They might remind you of how you used to love dancing or cooking. Starting small can help ease you back in. If you used to play guitar daily, for example, spend just 10 minutes strumming at first. This helps you avoid overwhelm while letting the fun return naturally.

12.4 Exploring New Interests

Quitting alcohol is a big change, so why not pair it with trying something completely new? It might be a sport you have never considered, such as badminton or rock climbing. Or a creative project like sewing, pottery, or photography. Trying new things can refresh your outlook, showing you that life has more to offer than just bars or parties.

Seek out free or low-cost classes in your community. Many libraries, local adult schools, or community centers offer beginner classes for crafts, fitness, or cooking. Attending these can lead to meeting people who share your new interest. That social connection helps replace drinking buddies with hobby buddies. Even if you do not stick with everything you try, the process itself can be exciting and keep you focused on personal growth.

12.5 Physical Activities and Outdoor Fun

One great way to fill time is with outdoor exercise or physical pursuits. This does not mean you must become a marathon runner. Simple activities like walking, biking, or gentle hiking can be very rewarding. Nature can calm the mind, and moving your body releases feel-good chemicals that help reduce stress.

If you prefer group settings, consider joining a casual sports league or a hiking club. You do not have to be an expert—many groups welcome beginners. The key is to find something you enjoy, not something that feels like a chore. Over time, this can become a new routine. Instead of hitting a bar after work, you might go for a walk in the park. This shift not only helps your sobriety but also improves physical health.

12.6 Volunteering and Giving Back

Using some of your free time to help others can bring a deep sense of purpose. Volunteering connects you with your community, makes you feel needed, and keeps you occupied with tasks that matter. There are many ways to volunteer: reading to children at a library, helping at an animal shelter, serving meals at a homeless center, or assisting in local clean-up events.

When you volunteer, you see life from a broader angle. You might meet people from different backgrounds, or learn new skills like event organization. This can shift your focus away from your own cravings and stress, reminding you that you can make a positive difference in the world. The personal satisfaction you get can serve as a strong motivator to remain sober.

12.7 Crafting a Weekly Schedule

Some women do best with a structured routine. If that sounds like you, try creating a simple schedule for your free hours. Map out your mornings, afternoons, and evenings with both responsibilities (like house chores) and leisure pursuits. This does not mean every minute must be filled. It is just a guideline to prevent aimless hours that might tempt you to drink out of boredom.

You might label blocks of time: "Walk in the neighborhood," "Read a novel," "Practice guitar," or "Volunteer at the community center." By giving your day a structure, you reduce the chance of drifting into old habits. You also get a sense of accomplishment when you see how many positive activities you complete each day. It is a reminder that your free time can be used in ways that support your goals instead of pulling you away from them.

12.8 Socializing Without Alcohol

One challenge is that many social activities revolve around drinking. You might have attended parties, gone to clubs, or met friends at a pub. Now that you are sober, you need alternatives. Here are some suggestions:

- **Coffee or Tea Meetups**: Invite friends to a local cafe instead of a bar.

- **Movie Nights at Home**: Stream a film or watch a classic DVD together. Provide snacks that do not involve alcohol.
- **Group Workouts**: Go to a yoga class or a dance fitness session with friends.
- **Board Game Parties**: These can be surprisingly fun. Ask everyone to bring a board or card game.
- **Picnics or Barbecues**: Focus on food and conversation, not on drinks. You can bring interesting non-alcoholic beverages, such as flavored sparkling waters or homemade fruit punches.

You might worry that friends who are used to drinking will find these options boring. But good friends will respect your choice and may even be curious about new ways to have fun. Over time, you might discover which friends are open-minded and which are not. This can be a tough lesson, but it also helps you form a circle of people who support your sober lifestyle.

12.9 Small Daily Rituals for Calm

Filling your free time does not always mean big activities or social events. Small daily rituals can be just as impactful. These might include:

- **Morning Gratitude**: Write or think of three things you appreciate before starting your day.
- **Afternoon Stretch Break**: Pause around midday to do a quick stretch or short breathing exercise.
- **Evening Calm-Down**: Light a scented candle, play soft music, and read something uplifting before bed.

These tiny steps help you build a sense of well-being without alcohol. By sprinkling such moments throughout your day, you keep your mind off cravings and remind yourself that a healthier, calmer life is within reach. Over time, these small rituals can become automatic, a steady backdrop to your sober journey.

12.10 Using Creativity for Personal Growth

Creative pursuits give your mind something fresh to focus on. This might include painting, writing, crafting, or even cooking. Each project becomes a way to channel energy you used to spend on drinking. When you start a creative project, you practice patience, problem-solving, and self-expression. These skills can also help you handle tough emotions or cravings.

You do not need to be a pro. Many creative activities are more about enjoying the process than producing a masterpiece. Some women take up simple do-it-yourself projects, like making candles or scrapbooking. Others try journaling daily, discovering that writing helps them sort out thoughts and feelings. You might even combine creativity with socializing, such as organizing a "craft night" with friends.

12.11 Exploring Educational Opportunities

Free time can also be an opportunity to learn. Maybe you always wanted to pick up a second language, study history, or learn coding. With online courses and tutorials, you can begin from the comfort of home. This not only keeps you busy but also feeds your mind. As you build new skills, your confidence grows.

Check local community colleges or adult learning centers for evening classes. Some are very affordable, and you might meet new, sober-minded friends in the process. Learning something new gives you a sense of progress and can open up future opportunities, whether for a career boost or just personal fulfillment.

12.12 Travel and Local Exploration

If you have the ability, consider short trips or local exploration. You do not have to go far or spend a fortune. Look up nearby parks, landmarks, or nature trails you have never visited. This can inject excitement into your free time and offer a change of scenery. Even a short drive to a neighboring town for the day can feel like a mini break.

While traveling, be mindful of triggers. Some people associate hotels or vacation settings with drinking. Plan ahead by bringing your own beverages (non-alcoholic) and filling your itinerary with activities that do not center on bars or parties. This might be hiking, visiting a museum, or trying local cuisines at eateries that focus on good food over alcohol. By exploring the world sober, you might find you remember your experiences more clearly and enjoy them more deeply.

12.13 Balancing Rest and Activity

Filling your free time does not mean you must stay busy every second. Rest is also vital. Some women feel guilty if they are not "productive" all the time. But relaxing can be healthy, provided you are not turning to old habits. A little bit of downtime can recharge your mind, making it easier to resist cravings when you get back to your daily routine.

Strike a balance. Set aside periods for rest, such as a quiet half-hour in the late afternoon. Use that time to lie down, breathe slowly, or listen to soothing music. The key is to keep your rest intentional, not simply zone out in a fog that leads to boredom and triggers. If you notice your mind drifting toward thoughts of having a drink, gently guide yourself to a calm activity like reading a few pages of a book.

12.14 Involving Loved Ones in Your New Activities

If you have children, a partner, or close friends, you can invite them to join your new pursuits. This can strengthen bonds and show them that fun does not require alcohol. For instance, you could plan a weekend arts-and-crafts session at home with your kids, teaching them simple painting or clay molding. Or you might suggest a family bike ride, exploring paths near your neighborhood. A partner might enjoy trying a new recipe with you in the kitchen, turning it into a shared project.

Involving loved ones can be tricky if they still drink. Be clear about your boundaries. Maybe you do not mind if they have a drink once in a while, but ask them not to do it around you during these new activities. Over time, your choice to remain sober may inspire them to cut back, too, or at least respect your environment.

12.15 Staying Open-Minded to Adjustments

You might try an activity for a few weeks and then realize it is not for you. That is okay. Part of filling free time is experimentation. Avoid judging yourself if you lose interest. Move on to something else that sparks your curiosity. The important thing is to keep learning what works best for you in this new stage of life.

Also, as you grow more confident in sobriety, your schedule might shift. Early on, you might need very structured daily plans, but later you might feel comfortable being more spontaneous. Allow yourself to adapt. The main goal is to stay engaged in life, enjoy your free hours, and keep your mind away from old habits that harm you.

12.16 Using Free Time for Self-Reflection

Some free time can be devoted to reflecting on your progress. You might set aside a quiet Sunday afternoon each month to note how many days you have stayed sober, how you handled triggers, and which activities brought you the most joy. This reflection can help you spot patterns. Maybe you find that gardening relaxes you more than anything else, or that certain social events feel too risky at this stage.

Use a journal or a digital planner to record these insights. Over time, you build a track record of personal growth. This can boost your confidence and show you that your life is indeed changing for the better. It is hard to see progress day by day, but looking back over a month or two can reveal big steps forward.

12.17 Conclusion of Chapter 12

Making better use of free time is a crucial part of staying sober. Boredom, loneliness, and restlessness can all lead to cravings if not managed. By filling your hours with activities that matter—whether creative, social, educational, or physical—you create a life that feels full. You no longer see free time as a dangerous zone but as a chance to do something meaningful.

This shift in how you spend your time can also rebuild your self-esteem. You prove to yourself that you are capable of living without alcohol, and that life can actually become richer and more interesting. Whether you rediscover old passions or start fresh with new hobbies, each moment you spend in a purposeful way is a victory. The sober life is not just about removing alcohol; it is about creating a space where healthier habits and real joy can grow.

Chapter 13: Handling Social Events Without Alcohol

13.1 Introduction: The Social Puzzle

Social events can be fun, but they can also be tricky when you have quit drinking. You might attend birthday parties, weddings, office outings, or holiday gatherings. In many of these situations, alcohol is present. You may see people toasting, pouring drinks, or handing out cocktails. If you used to drink at these events, it might feel odd to stand there without a glass in your hand. At first, you might worry that you will feel left out or pressured.

Yet, social events do not need to revolve around alcohol. This chapter will explore ways to enjoy parties, dinners, or group activities without feeling uncomfortable or out of place. You will find that these events can actually become more enjoyable when you stay clear-headed. Rather than avoiding gatherings out of fear, you can face them with the right mindset and plan.

13.2 Understanding the Social Setting

Before you attend any social event, think about what type of gathering it is. Some events, like office meetings or family lunches, might have little to no alcohol served. Others, like big parties or celebrations, might have a bar. Try to get details ahead of time:

- **Who will be there?** If you know the guest list includes heavy drinkers, you can prepare yourself.
- **Will alcohol be central?** Some parties are built around tasting wines or mixing cocktails. Others simply offer drinks as an option.
- **What are the main activities?** If the event centers on dancing, games, or food, you can focus on those. But if the main activity is drinking, you may have to decide whether to go at all.

Gathering this information helps you form a plan. You do not want to show up without a strategy, only to realize the entire evening revolves around alcoholic drinks.

13.3 Planning Ahead for Success

Once you know the nature of the event, make a plan. This plan can include:

1. **Arrival and Departure Times**
   If you suspect the party will ramp up in the later hours, consider arriving earlier and leaving before people get too rowdy. Or you might do the opposite—come later to minimize the time you spend around flowing drinks. You can also set a firm time to leave, so you are not stuck if things become too tempting.
2. **Non-Alcoholic Drinks**
   Think about what you will sip on. Sometimes, the host provides soft drinks or sparkling water. Other times, you might want to bring your own non-alcoholic drinks, especially if you are attending a potluck or casual gathering. Having a tasty option in hand can help you feel included.
3. **Transportation**
   Drive yourself or have a reliable ride. If you feel overwhelmed, you can leave without waiting for someone else to finish drinking. If you rely on a friend who plans to stay all night, you might be stuck.
4. **Support Buddy**
   If possible, bring someone who respects your decision not to drink. This person can be a friend, spouse, or even a coworker who is also avoiding alcohol. Having an ally there means you have someone to talk to and lean on if you feel uneasy.

Planning does not mean you assume the event will be unpleasant. It just means you have tools ready so you do not get caught off guard.

13.4 What to Say When Offered a Drink

One common worry is how to respond when people ask why you are not drinking. The simplest approach is a brief, polite answer. You do not need to give a full explanation or a long story. Some replies you can use:

- "No, thanks. I'm good with what I have."
- "I've decided not to drink tonight."
- "I'm driving."
- "I'm pacing myself—just water for me now."

Most people will not press further. If someone does push, you can repeat your statement or change the subject. If they still do not respect your boundary, it may say more about them than about you.

13.5 Handling Awkward or Pushy Individuals

Some people get uncomfortable when they see someone not drinking. They might tease or insist, "Just have one!" They could claim the event is "boring without alcohol." This can be annoying or stressful. A few tips:

- **Stay Calm**: Do not argue or get upset. Simply repeat that you are not drinking.
- **Redirect**: Shift focus to a different topic. For example, ask them about their job or a hobby.
- **Stand Your Ground**: If they keep pushing, you can respond with something firm like, "I'm not drinking, but I'd love to still enjoy the party with you. Tell me more about what you've been up to."

If someone continues to bother you, consider moving away to a different part of the room or talking to another guest. You do not owe them a detailed explanation. You are there to enjoy the event, not to defend your choice all night.

13.6 Finding Fun in Activities Besides Drinking

One reason people say they drink at parties is to loosen up or have fun. But there are many ways to enjoy yourself that do not involve alcohol:

1. **Focus on Conversations**
   Use your clear mind to have deeper, more meaningful chats. Ask people about their interests or experiences. You might learn interesting facts and build stronger connections.
2. **Join Games or Dancing**
   If there are party games, join in. Dancing can be a great stress release, too, even if you are sober. In fact, dancing sober lets you actually remember your moves and the laughter that goes with it.
3. **Enjoy the Food**
   Some events have great snacks or meals. Pay attention to flavors,

textures, and different dishes. You can savor these experiences instead of mindlessly gulping down drinks.

4. **Volunteer to Help**
   If the host is a friend, you can offer to help serve food, set up music, or tidy things. Staying busy in a productive way keeps your mind engaged and away from temptations.

By shifting your focus to the positive elements, you will find that parties have many dimensions beyond alcohol.

13.7 Setting Boundaries with Friends and Family

If you have friends or family members who drink often, you might find social gatherings challenging. You do not want to miss out, but you also do not want to be pressured. Boundaries help. For instance, if a friend hosts regular happy hours, you could say, "I'd love to see you, but can we pick a place that has other activities, like a coffee shop or a restaurant with non-alcoholic options?" If a relative insists on serving alcohol at every family meal, you might ask them politely if they can also have some special non-alcoholic options for you.

You might need to repeat these requests. Some people do not understand how important they are. Stay firm. Over time, people who truly respect you will make an effort to accommodate your choice.

13.8 Handling Celebrations and Big Events

Major events, like weddings or holiday parties, often involve toasts or group drinking. These can be tricky, but you can navigate them with a plan:

- **Toasts**: If everyone is raising a glass of champagne, you can lift a non-alcoholic beverage. Most guests will not even notice what is in your glass.
- **Holiday Gatherings**: If you visit relatives for a holiday, bring something you enjoy drinking, like a fancy sparkling cider. Offer it to others, too.
- **Weddings**: Some receptions feature an open bar, which can be tempting. Focus on the celebration itself—talk to people you have not seen in a

while, admire the decorations, or hit the dance floor. Step outside for fresh air if you feel overwhelmed.

Being sober at these events often means you remember the details clearly. You can truly share in the happiness of the occasion without hazy memories or regrets the next day.

13.9 Creating Your Own Social Activities

If you find traditional events too centered on alcohol, why not plan your own? Host gatherings that focus on something else, like:

- **Game Nights**: Invite friends for board games or card games. Provide fun snacks and mocktails (non-alcoholic mixed drinks).
- **Book Clubs**: Arrange a small group to discuss a chosen book each month. Serve tea or coffee.
- **Outdoor Adventures**: Plan a picnic, a hike, or a trip to a nature park with friends. Pack interesting sandwiches and fresh fruit drinks.
- **Movie Marathons**: Pick a theme, choose a few films, and enjoy them together. Serve popcorn and different flavored sodas.

By offering alcohol-free social options, you shape the environment to fit your needs. This also shows others that events can be lively and fun without alcohol. Over time, you might find more people joining in than you expected.

13.10 Dealing with Anxiety About Being Sober in Public

Some women feel anxious at the thought of attending social events without a drink to calm their nerves. They worry they will appear stiff or that they will not know how to interact. However, alcohol only masks social anxiety; it does not fix it. Learning to socialize sober is a skill that grows with practice.

One approach is to set small goals. For instance, decide you will talk to at least one new person at an event. Or promise yourself to stay for at least one hour before leaving. Each time you succeed, your confidence grows. You realize you can be witty, friendly, or warm without relying on alcohol.

You can also use relaxation methods before heading out. Take a few deep breaths, remind yourself of your reasons for quitting, and go in with a clear mind. Having a non-alcoholic drink in hand sometimes helps you feel less exposed, since many people simply want something to sip while chatting. Even if it is just water or a soft drink, it can ease the feeling of being empty-handed.

13.11 Knowing When to Leave

Not every event will go smoothly. Sometimes, people might start drinking more heavily, and the atmosphere may become tense or wild. If you feel uncomfortable or tempted, do not hesitate to leave. This is not rude. You have a right to protect your sobriety and peace of mind.

Have an exit strategy. Drive yourself, keep money for a taxi, or have a rideshare app ready. If someone asks why you are leaving early, a simple "I have an early morning" or "I need to get home" is enough. You do not owe anyone a long explanation. Leaving a situation that threatens your well-being is a sign of self-respect, not weakness.

13.12 Reflecting on Your Experience

After you attend a social event sober, take some time to think about how it went. Ask yourself:

- **What worked well?** Maybe bringing your own drinks helped or coming with a supportive friend made a difference.
- **What felt tough?** Did you feel pressure from certain people? Did a particular moment trigger cravings?
- **What can be improved next time?** If you stayed too long, perhaps you can leave earlier next time. If you forgot to bring a non-alcoholic option, you can remember in the future.

By reflecting, you learn from each event. Over time, you build a toolkit of successful strategies. This boosts your confidence and reduces anxiety about future gatherings.

13.13 Enjoying Clear-Headed Social Events

It might feel new or strange at first, but many women eventually find socializing without alcohol to be more satisfying. You remember conversations better, your mood stays more stable, and you avoid embarrassing situations. You can drive home safely without worrying about being impaired. The day after, you wake up feeling good instead of dealing with a hangover.

Being fully present also allows you to see which social connections are truly meaningful. Sometimes, when alcohol is removed, certain friendships fade because they were based on drinking. This can be sad, but it also clears room for more genuine bonds built on shared interests or mutual support. Your time becomes filled with deeper conversations and more honest laughter. You might even notice you have more energy to engage with others, making events more enjoyable.

13.14 Working with Hosts to Create a Sober-Friendly Space

If you are close to the person hosting the event, consider having a chat with them beforehand. You might say, "I do not drink anymore, but I really want to come and have fun. Could we make sure there are some non-alcoholic options, like club soda with lime or a fruit punch?" Many hosts will be happy to accommodate. Sometimes they do not realize how important it is to offer alternatives.

You could also suggest an interesting "mocktail" recipe or bring one yourself. For example, you can mix sparkling water with fresh berries, citrus slices, or herbs like mint. This creates a festive drink that does not involve alcohol. Other guests who might not drink much will likely appreciate it, too. By being proactive, you help shape the environment for everyone's benefit.

13.15 Traveling for Events

If you travel out of town for weddings, reunions, or other large gatherings, a little extra planning helps. Know which restaurants you will visit and see if they serve good non-alcoholic options. Pack your own small stash of sparkling water or a favorite soda for your hotel room. If you are staying with relatives who like to drink, politely mention your plan to remain sober. That way, they are less likely to push drinks on you.

Hotels sometimes offer happy hour deals or mini-bars in rooms. Request a room without a mini-bar or ask the staff to remove the alcohol. Some might raise an eyebrow, but many are used to such requests. Remember that your comfort matters. Reducing potential temptations can go a long way in helping you stay on track.

13.16 Staying Aware of Triggers

Even with careful planning, triggers can sneak up on you. A certain song might remind you of past party days. The sight of your old favorite drink might make your mouth water. Or you might feel a surge of stress if you see someone you once had conflicts with. Recognize these moments for what they are: passing temptations or reminders of old habits.

Use the methods you have learned so far—take a breath, distract yourself with another conversation, or step outside for a moment to clear your head. If you have an accountability partner, a quick text or call can help you refocus. Remind yourself why you quit drinking in the first place. This moment will pass, and you will be proud that you did not give in.

13.17 Conclusion of Chapter 13

Handling social events without alcohol is completely possible, even if it seems daunting at first. The key is to prepare in advance: know what kind of event it is, have a plan for what you will drink, figure out how to respond politely to offers, and decide how long you will stay. Over time, you will become more comfortable with sober socializing, and you may even start to prefer it.

By focusing on conversations, activities, and genuine connections, you will discover that events can be richer and more meaningful without alcohol. The clarity you gain will help you truly engage with others. You will leave gatherings feeling proud instead of guilty, rested instead of hungover, and strong instead of regretful. Social life becomes not a barrier to your new lifestyle, but a chance to grow and enjoy real friendships and experiences.

Chapter 14: Strategies for Bad Days

14.1 Introduction: Acknowledging Tough Times

Nobody goes through life without hitting tough days. These could be days when work feels overwhelming, family responsibilities pile up, or you simply wake up in a bad mood. In the past, you might have turned to alcohol for a quick escape from these down moments. Now that you are quitting, you need new ways to handle those emotional dips. The good news is, it can be done.

This chapter offers practical strategies to get you through rough patches without a drink. We will look at both immediate steps for when you feel panicked or upset, and longer-term changes that help reduce the frequency of bad days. Remember, a day that starts poorly does not need to end the same way. You have the power to shift your mindset and protect your sobriety.

14.2 Recognizing the Early Signs of a Bad Day

Bad days do not always hit suddenly. Sometimes, the signs start the night before—poor sleep, worrying thoughts, or conflict with someone close. Other times, you might notice physical cues like a tense jaw, tight shoulders, or a clenched stomach. If you catch these signals early, you can take preventative steps:

- **Mental Check-In**: Ask yourself, "Am I anxious or sad about something? Did something happen recently that is still bothering me?"
- **Physical Check-In**: Notice if your body feels stiff or uncomfortable. Sometimes, tension indicates you are carrying stress.
- **Environmental Check-In**: Did anything in your environment change? Perhaps you have a big deadline at work or a family event looming that is causing worry.

Identifying these signs can prevent a spiral. If you know a storm is coming, you can prepare a plan instead of feeling blindsided.

14.3 Immediate Relief Methods

When negative feelings first arise, it is helpful to have quick relief tools to stop them from spiraling:

1. **Deep Breathing**
   Try a short breathing exercise like inhaling for four counts, holding for four, and exhaling for four. This slows your heart rate and calms your mind.
2. **Grounding Exercise**
   Look around and name five things you see, four things you can touch, three things you hear, two things you smell, and one thing you taste. This technique shifts your focus from your worries to the present moment.
3. **Short Walk**
   If possible, step outside. Feel the air on your face, observe the sky, and listen to any sounds around you. Physical movement combined with fresh air can clear tension.
4. **Soothing Music or Sounds**
   Put on a calming tune, nature sounds, or even a playlist that lifts your mood. Close your eyes and let yourself tune into the music instead of your negative thoughts.

These immediate steps can bring a sense of calm, allowing you to think more clearly about the problem at hand.

14.4 Shifting Your Perspective

Bad days often worsen when your mind focuses on negative thoughts: "I can't handle this," or "Everything is going wrong." While you cannot simply flip a switch and feel great, you can shift your perspective a bit. Some tips:

- **Ask a Different Question**: Instead of "Why is everything awful?" ask, "What small step can I take to make things a bit better right now?"
- **Reframe Setbacks**: If you made a mistake at work, see it as a learning moment rather than a failure.
- **Practice Gratitude**: Write down a few things you still appreciate, even on a bad day. This might be a comfortable bed, a supportive friend, or a pet that brings you joy. Sometimes, noticing the good helps balance out the bad.

These small shifts might not erase all problems, but they can lighten the emotional load enough to keep you away from the urge to drink.

14.5 Distracting Yourself in Positive Ways

When a day feels overwhelming, one key strategy is healthy distraction. Rather than sitting in misery or grabbing a drink, fill your time with something else. This could be:

- **Creative Tasks**: Sketching, painting, writing in a journal, or cooking a new recipe.
- **Small Chores**: Tidying a drawer, organizing photos, or doing a quick clean-up. Seeing immediate results can lift your mood.
- **Light Entertainment**: Watching a comedy show or reading a short story. Laughter and mild escapism can reset your emotional state.
- **Reach Out**: Call or text a friend for a quick chat. Sometimes, just hearing someone else's voice can pull you out of a negative headspace.

The goal is not to ignore your problems permanently but to pause the emotional spiral. Once calmer, you can tackle issues with a clearer mind.

14.6 Using Your Support System

If you have set up a strong network (as discussed in Chapter 11), a bad day is exactly when to lean on it. Contact a trusted friend, family member, or accountability partner. Explain how you feel. You do not have to offer a perfect explanation—just say you are struggling and need someone to hear you out. Often, sharing your burden eases it.

If your support person is busy, try an online support forum. Post a short message about your day. People who have been through similar challenges can offer quick words of advice or simply let you know you are not alone. This feeling of connection can reduce the sense that your problems are too big to handle.

14.7 Making Small Adjustments to Your Routine

Some bad days happen because your routine has been disrupted. Maybe you skipped breakfast or stayed up too late the night before. Small adjustments can prevent little problems from turning into big ones:

- **Eat Regular Meals**: Hunger can make you irritable and amplify negative emotions.
- **Stay Hydrated**: Dehydration can affect your mood and energy levels.
- **Keep a Sleep Schedule**: Going to bed and waking up at consistent times supports emotional balance.
- **Include Breaks**: If your day is jam-packed, schedule brief pauses every couple of hours to breathe, stretch, or just sit quietly.

By looking after these basic needs, you make it less likely that a minor hassle will turn into a craving for alcohol.

14.8 Handling Stressful Situations Without Alcohol

Sometimes, a bad day is triggered by a specific event, like an argument with a loved one or a problem at work. In these cases, the temptation to drink can be strong because you want immediate relief. Instead, try:

1. **Address the Issue if Possible**
   Can you fix the problem by talking it out or sending an email to clarify misunderstandings? Taking proactive steps might reduce stress.
2. **Seek Advice**
   If you are unsure what to do, ask someone you trust, such as a mentor or counselor.
3. **Break the Situation into Parts**
   Focus on one aspect at a time. Overwhelm often comes from seeing the issue as one giant mess.

Alcohol might provide a brief escape, but the problem will still be there once you sober up. Dealing with it directly can bring genuine relief.

14.9 Unplugging from Negativity

Modern life can fill your mind with more stress than necessary. Checking the news too often, scrolling social media with its dramas, or engaging in heated online debates can darken your mood. On a bad day, consider stepping back from these sources of negativity:

- **Turn Off News Alerts**: You can always catch up later when you feel calmer.
- **Limit Social Media**: Set a timer to ensure you do not scroll endlessly.
- **Choose Positive Content**: Watch uplifting videos or read inspiring articles.
- **Mute or Unfollow Triggers**: If certain people or pages constantly upset you, distance yourself for the sake of your mental health.

This does not mean ignoring real-world issues forever, but a temporary break can shield you from extra negativity when you are already feeling low.

14.10 Self-Compassion and Kindness

On a bad day, people often beat themselves up. They might say, "I should be handling this better," or "I'm a mess." This harsh inner dialogue only adds to the pain. Practicing self-compassion involves treating yourself the way you would treat a dear friend. If your friend was having a bad day, you likely would not scold them. You would offer understanding and support.

- **Speak Kindly to Yourself**: Instead of "I'm failing," try "I'm going through a tough time, and I'll do what I can to get through it."
- **Acknowledge Your Effort**: Even if the day is rough, notice you are still trying. That effort deserves respect.
- **Forgive Slip-Ups**: If you snapped at someone, see it as a sign of stress, not a reflection of your entire character. Apologize if needed, then move on.

Self-compassion does not mean ignoring problems. It means facing them without adding extra layers of guilt or shame.

14.11 Physical Ways to Release Tension

Negative feelings can lodge themselves in your body. Activities that help release physical tension can brighten your mood:

1. **Stretching or Yoga-Like Movements**: No need for a fancy routine—just loosen tight muscles in your neck, shoulders, and back.
2. **Quick Exercise**: A short burst of physical activity, like jumping jacks or squats, can pump up endorphins.
3. **Massage or Self-Massage**: If you can, get a massage. If not, you can gently press and relax your own shoulders or use a simple device like a foam roller.
4. **Hand Tension Release**: Many of us hold tension in our hands. Clench your fists for a few seconds, then relax. Repeat several times to let stress flow out.

These methods do not solve the source of stress, but they make it more manageable by helping your body let go of some anxiety.

14.12 Checking Your Thoughts About Alcohol

On a bad day, it is easy to glamorize alcohol as a cure. You might think, "A drink will calm me down," or "I deserve a break from this misery." Challenge these thoughts with reality:

- **The Calm Is Temporary**: Alcohol might dull your feelings for an hour or two, but the stress or sadness usually returns stronger later.
- **New Problems Could Form**: Drinking can lead to poor decisions, arguments, or even more stress once you realize you broke your sober streak.
- **There Are Other Options**: You have a toolbox of skills—breathing, calling a friend, distraction, self-compassion, and more. It might not feel as instant, but it is healthier in the long run.

Remind yourself why you decided to quit. Picture how you want to feel tomorrow morning. That clear sense of purpose can help you push through.

14.13 Creating a Personal Bad Day Kit

Consider preparing a physical or digital "bad day kit" you can turn to when things get rough. It might include:

1. **Comfort Items**
   A soft blanket, a stress ball, or a small stuffed toy that gives you comfort.
2. **Positive Reminders**
   A list of reasons for quitting alcohol, encouraging quotes, or photos of loved ones.
3. **Distraction Tools**
   A favorite puzzle book, adult coloring pages, or a deck of cards.
4. **Calming Aids**
   A scented candle, lavender oil, or a calming playlist saved on your phone.
5. **Emergency Numbers**
   Contacts of friends, hotlines, or your counselor, in case you need urgent support.

Having these items in one place means you do not have to search for relief when you are already upset. You can grab your kit, find a quiet spot, and let the items guide you back to a calmer state.

14.14 Reaching Out for Professional Help When Needed

Sometimes, bad days cross a line into more severe moods—overwhelming sadness, constant anxiety, or thoughts of harming yourself. If you notice that these feelings linger for more than a few days or they intensify, it might be time to speak to a professional. You are not weak for seeking help. On the contrary, it shows courage.

A mental health counselor can offer therapy sessions. A doctor can evaluate whether medication could help stabilize your mood. If you feel unsafe, local hotlines or crisis numbers can provide immediate assistance. Remember, many individuals go through rough patches that need professional intervention. Accepting help early can prevent deeper problems down the road.

14.15 Building Resilience

Resilience is the ability to bounce back when life knocks you down. You build it over time by practicing the strategies mentioned here: self-care, support systems, problem-solving, and healthy thinking patterns. Each time you face a bad day without resorting to alcohol, you strengthen your resilience. You send your mind the message: "I can handle difficulties and stay sober."

Resilience also grows when you learn from your struggles. Maybe you discover you tend to have bad days after skipping meals or not sleeping enough. By adjusting those habits, you reduce future issues. Or you realize that talking to a certain friend calms you quickly, so you make a point of reaching out to them when you feel low. Over time, these lessons make you more adaptable and confident.

14.16 Reflecting and Moving Forward

At the end of a tough day, take a moment to reflect:

- **What Happened?** Summarize the day's main stress points or triggers.
- **How Did You Respond?** Which tools did you use? Did you reach out to someone, take a walk, or do a breathing exercise?
- **What Will You Keep in Mind for Next Time?** Maybe you realized that journaling helps you more than you expected, or that skipping social media improved your mood.

By reflecting, you see that even on bad days, you are learning and growing. You do not have to ignore the negative feelings. Instead, you handle them in a healthier way than before. This process of noticing, coping, and learning helps you refine your approach over time.

14.17 Conclusion of Chapter 14

Bad days happen. They are part of life. The difference now is that you do not have to reach for alcohol as the solution. You have alternative methods—breathing exercises, supportive connections, planned distractions, and a kinder way of speaking to yourself. By using these strategies, you transform a rough day into a manageable one. You also protect your sobriety and continue building the life you want.

Rather than letting a bad mood become an excuse to relapse, see it as a test that helps you grow stronger. Each time you pass that test, you gain self-trust. You learn that negative feelings are temporary waves, not permanent conditions. By the next day, your outlook might improve, or you might find a fresh perspective that was not visible before. Through consistent practice, you will see that staying sober is not only possible during smooth times but also during the stormy ones. And that realization is a major milestone in your path toward lasting change.

With the tools from this chapter, you can face tough moments without losing sight of your goals. In the upcoming chapters, we will continue examining ways to stay on track, move past slip-ups, and maintain the progress you have worked so hard to achieve. For now, remember that even on the darkest days, you have the power to choose a healthier way forward—one that keeps you free from alcohol.

Chapter 15: Sticking to New Habits

15.1 Introduction: From Initial Change to Long-Term Commitment

Deciding to quit drinking and taking the first steps are major victories. Yet, one challenge remains: turning these positive actions into permanent habits. Many women find that the first few weeks or months can be full of enthusiasm. After that, motivation might fade. Old routines may start sneaking back, making you wonder if you can keep up your new behaviors for the long run.

In this chapter, we will discuss how to make these changes stick. We will explore practical methods to maintain the new rhythms in your daily life. Whether you have been sober for a few weeks or a few months, these strategies will help you stay consistent and overcome the dips in motivation that can threaten your progress. You have already done a lot of work; now let us look at how to make these changes a true part of your life story.

15.2 Why Habits Matter More Than Willpower Alone

You may think that willpower is the only thing you need to stay away from alcohol. Certainly, determination is important. But relying solely on raw determination can be tiring. If you have a stressful day or feel low on energy, your willpower might drop. That is when old habits have a chance to creep back.

Building new habits, however, makes good choices feel automatic. A habit is an action you do without much conscious thought because you have repeated it so often. For instance, brushing your teeth at night likely feels like second nature. You do not wake up each morning debating if you should do it. Similarly, you can get to a point where pouring a non-alcoholic drink at dinner or going for a quick walk after work is just part of your routine.

When healthy activities become ingrained, you do not have to struggle with decisions over and over. This saves mental energy and helps you stay sober even on days when stress is high or your mood is off. That is the true power of habit—creating an internal system that guides you, rather than always leaning on determination.

15.3 Setting Clear Goals and Breaking Them Down

To stick with new habits, it helps to set clear goals. Vague aims like "I want to stay sober" can be overshadowed by daily temptations. But a specific, measurable goal keeps your focus. For example:

- "I will remain alcohol-free for the next 30 days."
- "I will attend one support meeting each week."
- "I will replace my usual evening drink with a cup of herbal tea."

Once you have a clear goal, break it down into smaller steps if needed. For instance, if your aim is to avoid alcohol at home, start by removing all bottles from your fridge. Then buy a variety of non-alcoholic drinks you enjoy, so you do not feel deprived. Set a routine—perhaps each evening, you will brew a pot of tea or mix sparkling water with fruit. This step-by-step approach makes it easier to stay on track.

15.4 Anchoring Habits to Existing Routines

One effective way to form lasting habits is to tie them to routines you already have. For example, if you normally watch TV for 30 minutes before bed, you could decide to do a quick stretch or relaxation exercise right afterward. That way, the new action becomes part of a familiar rhythm. Another example might be to take a brisk walk after dinner each night, right before washing the dishes. By placing the walk between dinner and dishes, it becomes a natural part of the evening flow.

Attaching a new behavior to an existing habit is called "habit stacking." It reduces the mental load of remembering to do something new. You are less likely to skip it when it is linked to a routine you rarely miss.

15.5 Tracking and Celebrating Small Victories

Monitoring your progress helps you stay mindful and motivated. You could keep a small notebook or an app where you check off days you stay sober or complete certain tasks. For instance, if your goal is to walk for 20 minutes each day instead of drinking, mark each successful day on a calendar. Over time, seeing those marks add up can be encouraging. It shows how far you have come, even if you do not always feel it day by day.

You can also give yourself small treats or signs of recognition when you reach a milestone. For example, if you go a month without drinking, treat yourself to a new book or something that brings you pleasure. These small rewards help lock in the idea that positive actions lead to positive outcomes. They keep the new habits fresh and remind you that your effort matters.

15.6 Staying Flexible with Your Habits

Life changes, and so do schedules. If you have a rigid plan—for example, you must always walk at 7:00 a.m.—what happens when you travel or have an early appointment? You might skip the walk and end up feeling like you failed, which can hurt motivation. Instead, keep your routines flexible. If you cannot walk at 7:00, maybe you walk at noon or after dinner. The key is to find a time that works, rather than giving up entirely.

Similarly, be flexible with the type of activity. If your usual plan is a 30-minute walk, but it is raining hard one day, you could do a short indoor workout instead. Being adaptable helps you keep the habit going regardless of small disruptions.

15.7 Dealing with Habit Fatigue

Habit fatigue is when you get tired of doing the same thing repeatedly. It can happen with healthy routines, too. If you find your morning exercise becoming dull or your evening non-alcoholic beverage no longer feels refreshing, it is time for a small change. This does not mean giving up the habit, but you can tweak it:

- **Try a new route for your walk**
- **Pick a different flavor of tea**
- **Switch up your usual reading spot**
- **Invite a friend to join you in your routine**

Making small adjustments keeps your habits from turning stale, which in turn keeps you engaged. Variety can help you stick with the overall goal.

15.8 Overcoming Plateaus

A plateau is a period where you stop seeing progress or feel stuck in a rut. Maybe you stopped drinking months ago, and you feel stable, but you are starting to question why you are still following certain routines, like frequent support meetings. You might think, "I'm fine now. Do I need to continue?" Plateaus can tempt you to ease up on the very routines that protect your sobriety.

Instead of stopping, use a plateau as a sign to reflect on what you have achieved and where you want to go next. Maybe it is time to challenge yourself by adding a new health goal, like improving your nutrition or learning a relaxing skill. Or perhaps you can offer help to others who are quitting, which may bring fresh motivation. Plateaus are not dead ends; they are signals to review, refresh, and keep growing.

15.9 The Role of Positive Self-Talk

How you talk to yourself matters. If you keep criticizing yourself for the smallest slip, you chip away at your confidence. On the other hand, positive self-talk supports your new habits. For instance, if you catch yourself thinking, "I'm so weak for even wanting a drink," challenge that thought. A balanced approach might be, "I'm doing well overall. A craving is just a reminder of my old pattern, and I have the power to handle it."

Developing a kinder internal dialogue can make a big difference in whether you stick with your habits. Encourage yourself the way you would encourage a friend. Remind yourself why these changes matter and how far you have already come.

15.10 Peer Accountability and Community Support

We discussed the value of a support system in Chapter 11. Here, it is worth noting how accountability can cement new habits. Maybe you have an accountability buddy who messages you each morning, asking if you have done your daily exercise or stayed away from alcohol. Or perhaps you check in with an online group once a week to report your progress.

Knowing that someone else is aware of your goals can boost your dedication. You feel you are not alone, and you also know someone will notice if you stray. This sense of shared responsibility can provide an extra push on days you do not feel like keeping up with your routines.

15.11 Balancing Self-Discipline with Self-Care

Sticking to new habits requires a degree of discipline, but it should not turn into punishing yourself. If you are too strict, you might burn out or resent your own routines. A healthier approach is to see your habits as acts of self-care. You are not forcing yourself; you are nurturing yourself.

For example, preparing a healthy meal at home instead of ordering alcoholic drinks and snacks is not just about denying yourself. It is about choosing foods that make you feel better and keep you on track. When you reframe your habits as caring gestures instead of harsh rules, you are more likely to stay motivated for the long term.

15.12 Knowing Your Personal Motivation

Everybody has unique reasons for quitting. Some do it for health, others for family, and still others for financial reasons. Write down your personal motivations and keep them in a place you see often—a note on your phone, a piece of paper on the fridge, or a small card in your wallet. When your new habits feel tough, look at this list. It reminds you of the bigger picture.

You might include statements like:

- "I want to have more energy to spend time with my children."
- "I want to save money for something special."
- "I want to protect my health and feel better each day."
- "I want to keep a clear mind for my work and my relationships."

These motivations act like a compass, guiding you back to the right path whenever you feel lost or tempted.

15.13 Planning for Busy or Stressful Periods

Life has busy seasons—maybe a major project at work or a family event that takes all your attention. During these times, it is easy to let healthy routines slip. Before a busy period arrives, think of how you will keep your habits alive. Perhaps you switch to shorter exercise sessions, make quick healthy meals in bulk, or attend an online support group if you cannot go in person.

Adjusting to life's pace is crucial. By planning ahead, you avoid the trap of "I'm too busy, so I guess I'll just drop my good habits." Instead, you carry a lighter version of them. Once the busy period ends, you can return to your normal routine without having to start from scratch.

15.14 Rewarding Yourself the Healthy Way

In the past, you might have used alcohol as a reward: "I had a rough day, so I deserve a drink." Now, you need different ways to honor your efforts. Healthy rewards can be simple yet meaningful:

- **Buy Yourself a Small Item You Have Been Eyeing**: It could be a scented candle, a new journal, or a cozy blanket.
- **Enjoy a Relaxing Activity**: Maybe a warm bath with bath salts or a home-based foot soak.
- **Plan a Free Treat**: Such as a quiet afternoon reading a fun book, or a scenic walk by a lake.
- **Mark Your Achievements**: Write down every small milestone, like "10 days sober" or "1 week of morning walks," and celebrate by telling a friend or family member who supports you.

Rewards do not have to be fancy or expensive. The point is to reinforce your positive behavior with something that feels good but does not pull you back into unhealthy territory.

15.15 Handling Criticism from Others

As you keep your new habits, some people might criticize or tease you. They may say you are overdoing it or that you used to be more "fun" when you drank. Such comments can sting. But remember that you are doing this for your well-being. If others cannot accept that, it is not your job to please them at the cost of your health.

You can respond politely or keep your boundaries firm. A calm reply might be, "I'm feeling better than ever, so this is what works for me." By standing your ground, you show self-respect. Over time, those who truly care will likely come around and realize how serious you are about these positive changes.

15.16 Reviewing and Updating Your Habits Regularly

Once a month or so, take time to review how your new habits are going. Ask yourself:

1. **What is working well?** Maybe the morning walk is still helpful.
2. **What is feeling stale or hard?** Perhaps you are bored with the same workout routine.
3. **Is there any routine I have accidentally dropped?** If so, decide whether to bring it back or replace it with something better.
4. **Have my goals changed?** Sometimes, you start with a goal of staying sober. Then you might add a goal of eating better or improving sleep.

By reviewing, you keep your habits current with your life. This periodic check-in prevents you from drifting off track without noticing.

15.17 Conclusion of Chapter 15

Sticking to new habits is the bridge between a short-term fix and a lasting change. You have already shown courage by quitting alcohol, and now you are focusing on the routines that keep you stable and strong. Rather than relying on sheer determination every day, you are weaving healthier actions into the fabric of your normal life.

You do this through goal-setting, flexible schedules, celebration of small wins, and a strong sense of personal motivation. You allow yourself to adapt when circumstances shift, instead of giving up at the first sign of trouble. Over time, these habits become part of who you are—a person who cares for her mind and body, a person who can face stress without turning to a drink.

Chapter 16: Understanding Setbacks

16.1 Introduction: The Reality of Slip-Ups

Life rarely goes in a straight line. Even with solid habits and strong resolve, a setback can occur. This might look like having a drink after several months of sobriety or falling back into old patterns for a week. Some women feel deep shame when this happens. They worry that they have lost all progress and might as well give up.

The truth is, a setback does not erase all your efforts. It is an event that can happen on the path to long-term change. What matters most is how you respond. Will you let it define you, or will you learn from it and carry on? In this chapter, we explore what setbacks are, why they happen, and how you can bounce back stronger. Accepting that slip-ups can be part of the process lets you plan for them without losing hope.

16.2 Identifying Different Types of Setbacks

A setback can take many forms. Not all are as simple as picking up a drink. Here are a few examples:

1. **Full Relapse**: Going back to a pattern of regular drinking for days or weeks, possibly neglecting other areas of life.
2. **One-Time Slip**: Having a single drink or a short binge, then realizing you need to stop immediately.
3. **Emotional Backslide**: Feeling the same guilt, anxiety, or negative thoughts you had when drinking, even if you do not actually pick up a drink.
4. **Replacing Alcohol with Another Unhealthy Habit**: Sometimes, a person might quit drinking but start overusing food, gambling, or another vice.

Recognizing the type of setback helps you decide what actions to take. A single slip may need a swift corrective measure, while a full relapse may call for deeper intervention.

16.3 Why Setbacks Happen

Setbacks can arise for many reasons. Some common triggers include:

- **High Stress**: Ongoing problems at work, conflict at home, or financial worries can push someone to seek relief in old ways.
- **Strong Emotions**: Sadness, anger, or loneliness might lead to a moment of weakness.
- **Overconfidence**: After a period of sobriety, a person might think, "I have this under control. One drink cannot hurt."
- **Sudden Changes**: A big life event like moving, a job loss, or the end of a relationship can unsettle your routines.
- **Environmental Triggers**: Being around old drinking buddies or visiting a familiar bar might spark temptation.

By understanding these causes, you can see that a setback is not just a personal flaw. Often, it is a response to a situation or feeling that you have not fully learned to handle yet.

16.4 The Emotional Effects of a Slip-Up

A slip-up often brings a wave of negative emotions—shame, guilt, anger at oneself, or fear that others will judge you. These feelings can be so strong that a woman might decide she has already failed, so continuing to drink does not matter. This kind of thinking can lead to a bigger relapse.

However, it is crucial to remember that one slip does not define you. Those uncomfortable emotions are signals that something went wrong. Rather than letting them crush you, you can use them as motivation. Acknowledge that you feel upset, then ask, "What can I do to correct this and prevent it from happening again?" That shift from shame to problem-solving is key to moving forward.

16.5 The Difference Between Lapse and Relapse

Some professionals distinguish between a "lapse" and a "relapse." A lapse is a single slip—a brief return to drinking. A relapse is a full return to old behaviors over a longer period. This distinction matters because it changes how you respond.

- **Lapse**: Often can be managed by recognizing it quickly, seeking help, and making immediate adjustments to your plan.
- **Relapse**: May require more intensive steps, such as revisiting a support program, possibly seeking professional counseling again, or renewing your commitment to daily sober routines.

By calling a single slip a lapse instead of a relapse, you can reduce panic and handle it in a level-headed way.

16.6 First Steps After a Slip-Up

If you find yourself in a slip-up situation, here are immediate actions you can take:

1. **Stop Drinking Right Away**: Pour out any remaining alcohol. Distance yourself from the environment that led to it.
2. **Tell Someone You Trust**: Admitting it to a friend, counselor, or accountability partner reduces shame. They can offer support and advice.
3. **Reflect on the Trigger**: Think about what specifically made you pick up a drink. Was it stress, anger, or an unexpected event?
4. **Return to Basics**: Revisit the routines that helped you stay sober in the first place—support meetings, healthy distractions, or daily checklists.
5. **Be Kind to Yourself**: Rather than beating yourself up, remember that you have the power to learn from this.

Acting quickly and honestly is the best way to prevent a slip from spiraling into a complete relapse.

16.7 Updating Your Plan

A setback indicates that something in your plan might need adjusting. Maybe you need more frequent contact with a sponsor or accountability buddy. Perhaps your stress levels are high, suggesting you need better stress management methods. You might also need to avoid certain places or people for a while.

Update your plan by writing down what went wrong and what changes you will make. Consider these questions:

- **Did I notice warning signs but ignore them?**
- **Did I fail to use a coping skill when stress peaked?**
- **Do I need to adjust my environment to remove temptations?**
- **Should I add or change a support group?**
- **Are there new challenges in my life I did not account for?**

By refining your plan, you are less likely to repeat the same mistake.

16.8 Learning from Each Setback

One of the most powerful ways to handle setbacks is to view them as lessons. Ask yourself:

1. **What was the sequence of events?** Identify the chain of thoughts or situations that led to the slip.
2. **Which coping strategies worked, and which did not?** Maybe you tried calling a friend but waited too long, or perhaps you never used the relaxation methods you know.
3. **How can I handle a similar situation in the future?** Come up with a concrete action you will take if the same trigger occurs again.

Learning from a slip transforms it from a failure into a stepping stone. Over time, you become more resilient because you understand yourself and your triggers better.

16.9 Watching Out for Self-Pity or Self-Punishment

After a setback, two extreme emotional responses might pop up:

- **Self-Pity**: Feeling sorry for yourself, telling yourself that everything is hopeless and that you are doomed to fail.
- **Self-Punishment**: Berating yourself harshly, believing you deserve bad outcomes because of your lapse.

Both can push you further away from your goal of staying sober. Self-pity can lead to giving up, while self-punishment can lower your self-esteem. A better approach is balanced self-reflection: "I made a mistake, I regret it, but I am capable of doing better next time." This mindset keeps you accountable without tearing you down.

16.10 Using Professional Help for Major Relapses

If you have had a full relapse, or if your slip-ups keep repeating despite your best efforts, it might be time to seek professional help again. This could include:

- **Going Back to Counseling**: Even a few sessions can help reset your mindset.
- **Inpatient or Outpatient Programs**: If the relapse is severe, a structured environment may help you regain stability.
- **Medication**: In some cases, a doctor might recommend medicines that reduce cravings or help manage mood issues tied to alcohol use.
- **Therapeutic Groups**: Some groups focus specifically on relapse prevention, teaching new coping skills for people who have slid back into old habits.

Seeking help is not admitting defeat; it is an active choice to protect yourself. Many individuals go through multiple phases of care before achieving stable, lasting change.

16.11 Communication with Family and Friends

A setback can affect not just you, but also the people around you—especially if they have been cheering you on. Family members might feel worried or disappointed. Friends might not know how to react. The best approach is honest communication. You can say something like, "I had a slip, but I am taking steps to correct it. I appreciate your support. I am not giving up."

By being open, you maintain trust. You also signal that you are serious about getting back on track. Loved ones might offer extra help during this time, such as being with you more often or helping you avoid risky situations until you feel strong again. Hiding a relapse often leads to more guilt and isolation, which can worsen the situation.

16.12 Keeping a Balanced Perspective

It is easy to blow a setback out of proportion and feel like everything is ruined. Remember, you are still the person who made a commitment to quit, and you succeeded for a certain period. One lapse does not erase the progress you have built. Think of all the lessons you have gained along the way: new coping skills, healthier relationships, a better understanding of your triggers, and more.

By keeping a balanced perspective, you see the slip in context. Yes, it is serious, but it is also one part of a bigger story. You can pick yourself up and keep going. The time and effort you invested in staying sober do not vanish because of a bad evening or a challenging week.

16.13 Rebuilding Self-Trust

After a slip-up, you might feel you cannot trust yourself. You promised you would not drink, and then you did. Regaining self-trust starts with small steps:

- **Honesty**: Acknowledge what happened, without excuse or denial.
- **Consistency**: Follow through on little promises you make to yourself, like attending a meeting or doing a daily check-in.
- **Patience**: Realize self-trust does not return overnight. Each day you stick to your plan is a day you rebuild confidence.
- **Self-Respect**: Recognize that one mistake does not define your entire character.

As you keep moving forward, you will find your self-confidence grows again. Each sober day is another example of your ability to choose a better path.

16.14 Adjusting Goals and Expectations

Sometimes, a setback reveals that your goals might have been too strict or your timeline too short. If you told yourself you had to be perfect from day one, any slip might feel like a total failure. Instead, adjust your expectations. Aim for steady improvement rather than perfection. Celebrate your sober days and learn from the days you struggle.

For instance, if you realized daily support meetings are too frequent to maintain, maybe you shift to a few times a week. If that remains consistent, it is more effective than a strict plan you cannot keep. By tailoring your goals to be realistic, you reduce the chance of feeling overwhelmed.

16.15 Returning to Healthy Habits

A setback sometimes leads people to abandon other healthy routines. You might stop exercising or start eating poorly, thinking, "I already messed up, so why bother?" Catch yourself if this occurs. Do not let one area of your life falling off track drag down every other area. Instead, reaffirm the healthy habits that you had.

- **Go back to your standard grocery list if you slipped into buying junk food**
- **Restart short workouts if you stopped them**
- **Return to the bedtime routine that helped you get good sleep**

Getting these routines back in place can stabilize your mood and give you a sense of control, making it easier to refocus on staying sober.

16.16 Telling Your Story Honestly

One of the strongest ways to handle a setback is to talk about it. If you attend support groups or have a mentor, sharing your slip can feel vulnerable at first. But honesty not only frees you from secrecy, it can also inspire others. People in the same boat understand how easy it is to trip up. By telling them what happened and what you learned, you show that setbacks can be faced rather than hidden.

You may also discover that other people have stories of relapse or slip-ups. Hearing how they recovered can offer fresh ideas. This shared experience fosters empathy and can strengthen your commitment to try again. People rarely judge you as harshly as you fear, especially in communities built around mutual support.

16.17 Conclusion of Chapter 16

Setbacks, whether a single slip or a longer relapse, do not have to spell the end of your efforts. They are signs that something in your plan or environment needs revisiting. By acting fast, being honest, and learning from the event, you can stand up again. A lapse is not the same as failure; it is an opportunity to understand yourself better and refine your strategies.

The key is to avoid letting one bad moment turn into a permanent backward step. You have come too far for that. A slip does not negate the sober days you have already achieved. By accepting the reality that slip-ups can happen and preparing for them, you become more resilient. You gain insight into your triggers and strengthen your resolve to keep going.

In upcoming chapters, we will discuss building self-respect and looking ahead to a brighter future without alcohol. We will also explore how you might support other women who are going through the same process. For now, remember that every setback carries the seed of a stronger comeback. You can use this as a stepping stone on your path to a lasting, healthier life free from alcohol.

Chapter 17: Building Self-Respect

17.1 Introduction: The Importance of Liking Yourself

Self-respect is not just a pleasant feeling; it is a strong force that can change your actions and your outlook on life. When you respect yourself, you believe you deserve good treatment, healthy relationships, and real happiness. For many women who have quit drinking or are working on it, self-respect can be the missing piece that helps them stay firm. Without self-respect, you might slip into patterns of shame, guilt, or self-doubt, all of which can make it harder to remain sober.

In this chapter, we will look at what self-respect means, why it matters for women who used alcohol as a crutch, and how you can build it in day-to-day life. We will cover practical ways to deal with negativity, both from within and from the outside world. Our goal is to show you that self-respect is not some fancy concept but a direct path to feeling better about who you are and the choices you make.

17.2 Defining Self-Respect in Basic Terms

Self-respect means you see yourself as worthy of kindness, care, and fairness. It is different from arrogance or thinking you are better than others. Instead, it is a balanced view of your own value as a person. When you have self-respect, you set limits on how others treat you. You also tend to make wiser decisions that protect your well-being.

Some people confuse self-respect with self-esteem. While they overlap, you can think of self-esteem as how you feel about your abilities, like how well you do at work or in social settings. Self-respect, on the other hand, is a deeper sense of worth. Even if you make mistakes, you can still hold onto self-respect, because it is about seeing that you matter, no matter what.

17.3 Why Women Struggle with Self-Respect After Drinking Problems

Many women who have had issues with drinking also deal with shame or guilt. They might blame themselves for hurting loved ones, losing money, or damaging their health. Over time, these thoughts can eat away at any sense of self-worth. Some women also face criticism from society or family, which can intensify the feeling that they do not deserve kindness or success.

These emotional blows make it hard to stand strong in self-respect. Instead, a woman might think, "I made so many mistakes, so I am not worth much." This attitude can lead to further harm, such as going back to alcohol or staying in unhealthy relationships. Reversing this mindset requires effort and a clear plan, but it is entirely possible. You can accept your past without letting it define your future.

17.4 Uncovering Past Hurts That Block Self-Respect

Sometimes, the root of low self-respect is not just about drinking. It might go back to childhood experiences, harmful words from parents, or traumatic events. If a girl grows up being told she is not good enough or feels responsible for family problems, she might carry those beliefs into adulthood. Drinking can become a way to numb that pain.

To move forward, you might need to explore these past hurts. This does not mean getting stuck in them forever. It simply means acknowledging they exist, understanding how they shaped you, and deciding they no longer have power over you. A counselor or therapist can be helpful here, offering tools to process old hurts so they do not keep controlling your sense of self.

17.5 Replacing Negative Thoughts with Balanced Views

One step toward self-respect is changing the internal messages you tell yourself. Many women with a history of drinking problems fall into negative self-talk. They might say, "I always fail," or "I am weak." To rebuild self-respect, you can practice catching these thoughts and replacing them with more balanced or positive statements.

For example, if you catch yourself thinking, "I cannot handle stress without a drink," pause and replace it with, "I handled stress yesterday by going for a walk, and I can do it again." If you think, "No one cares about me," you might replace it with, "Some people do care, even if I have had strained relationships. I can work on improving those connections now."

This shift in thinking will not happen overnight. It takes repeated practice, much like training a muscle. Over time, your brain will get used to the new, kinder messages. As a result, your sense of self-respect grows.

17.6 The Power of Physical and Mental Boundaries

Respecting yourself also means setting boundaries with others. This includes deciding which actions are okay and which are not. For instance, if you have a friend who always pressures you to drink, you can tell them kindly but firmly that you are not drinking anymore. If they ignore your requests or mock you, you have the right to limit your contact with them, at least until you feel more stable in your sobriety.

You might also need mental boundaries. This means stopping yourself from dwelling on thoughts that tear you down. If you notice a spiral of self-blame or shame, you can direct your focus elsewhere—perhaps on a constructive task, a calming activity, or by reading something uplifting. Each time you enforce these boundaries, you signal to yourself that your well-being matters.

17.7 Practical Exercises to Build Self-Respect

Below are some actions you can try in daily life to strengthen self-respect:

1. **Write Down Three Good Qualities About Yourself**
   Do this every morning or evening. It might feel silly at first, but it trains your mind to look for strengths instead of flaws.
2. **Practice Small Acts of Kindness to Yourself**
   This could be preparing a healthy meal, resting when tired, or letting yourself have some quiet time to read or do a hobby you like.
3. **Speak Your Needs Out Loud**
   Each day, identify one need you have—like a break from a stressful chore or help with a project—and ask someone you trust for support. This reminds you that your needs are valid.
4. **Say "No" When Needed**
   If someone asks you to do something that drains you or clashes with your health goals, practice saying a simple but firm no.

5. **Stand Tall and Look People in the Eye**
   Body language affects how you feel about yourself. Holding your head up can make you feel more confident inside.

17.8 Handling Criticism from Others

Sometimes, people around you might not understand your path. They may say hurtful things, whether intentional or not. It is key to remember that their words do not define you. If criticism is valid, learn from it. If it is just mean or based on ignorance, let it go. Dwelling on every negative remark will only drain your self-respect.

One technique is to remind yourself that everyone has opinions, but not all opinions matter the same. A counselor once suggested rating a critic's importance on a scale of 1 to 10. If the critic is someone you respect who knows you well, their opinion might be a 9 or 10, worth considering. If the critic is a random stranger or someone who has a history of unhelpful remarks, their opinion might be a 2 or 3, less significant in shaping how you see yourself.

17.9 Stepping Away from Toxic Relationships

An important part of building self-respect is stepping away from relationships that sap your confidence. Toxic relationships can be romantic, platonic, or even family ties. Signs include constant belittling, manipulation, or an expectation that you keep giving while receiving little support in return. You deserve better. Breaking free might be tough, but staying in a damaging dynamic can slow or block your progress in sobriety.

Leaving a toxic relationship might mean limiting contact, seeking legal help if safety is an issue, or ending the relationship altogether. This does not mean you hate the person; it means you are protecting yourself. Over time, as you surround yourself with healthier connections, your sense of self-respect will strengthen. You will also find it easier to stick to your decision to not drink, because you are no longer in an environment that pushes you toward old habits.

17.10 Affirming Your Past Achievements and Skills

One way to counter negative beliefs is to recall things you have done well in life, whether before or during your quitting phase. Maybe you succeeded at a past job, raised caring children, or learned a skill like painting or writing. These achievements show that you can handle challenges and produce good results.

Make a list of your skills and past successes. Refer to it when you start doubting your abilities. This helps you see that, yes, you may have stumbled at times, but you have also done many things right. You are not defined by your slip-ups.

17.11 Expanding Your Horizons with New Goals

Building self-respect can also mean expanding your vision for what is possible. If you have been sober for a while, you might have more time, energy, or mental clarity. Consider using that space to try new activities or work toward a dream. Maybe you want to start a small business, learn a musical instrument, or help your community in a volunteer role.

Each time you stretch beyond your comfort zone, you prove to yourself that you are capable. You form new identities that are not tied to alcohol or the problems it caused. This growth leads to a stronger sense of worth. When you see yourself achieving new things, you start to think, "I am really building a life I can respect."

17.12 Keeping Promises to Yourself

A powerful way to grow self-respect is to follow through on promises you make to yourself. These can be small, like waking up 15 minutes earlier for a quick walk, or larger, like attending a regular support meeting. Each time you keep a self-promise, you send the message, "I am a person who does what she says." This builds trust in yourself. If you break a promise, do not panic; note what got in the way and try again.

Over time, these small fulfillments add up. You will start to see yourself as someone who is reliable, even if the rest of the world feels unstable. This sense of self-reliance is key to staying sober because you will rely less on outside substances or people for reassurance.

17.13 Celebrating Personal Growth

When you reach milestones, such as a certain number of sober days or accomplishing something meaningful, it is good to recognize it. That does not mean throwing a huge party or going overboard. It can be a simple acknowledgment like writing in a journal, "Today marks six months without a drink, and I feel proud." You might treat yourself to a small, meaningful gift or take a relaxing outing to mark the moment.

These small acknowledgments reinforce the idea that your efforts matter. They show that you are willing to see your own worth. If you are in a support group, you can share your progress there, knowing that others will understand how much it means.

17.14 Seeking Role Models Who Demonstrate Self-Respect

Look for people who carry themselves with quiet confidence—women who treat others well but do not let themselves get walked on. They might be in your circle of friends, your workplace, or even public figures. Observe how they handle conflicts or setbacks. Notice how they say no when they need to, or how they calmly stand up for themselves.

You do not need to copy their entire personality. But seeing real examples of self-respect in action can inspire you. It shows you that it is not just theory; it is possible to live with dignity and calm strength. Sometimes, you can even reach out to these role models for advice, if the situation allows. They might have insights into how they built their sense of worth and how they handle negative pushback.

17.15 Fighting Comparison Traps

Comparing yourself to others can erode self-respect fast. You might see someone who has never had a drinking problem and think, "They are so much better than me." Or, you might compare your path of quitting to someone else's, noticing they had an "easier" time. This kind of thinking can leave you feeling inferior.

In reality, each person has a different background, set of challenges, and resources. Instead of comparing, focus on your own path. Remember that you have overcome unique obstacles and that your pace is your own. If you see someone doing well, let it inspire you rather than bring you down. If they can do it, that means it is possible for others, too.

17.16 How Self-Respect Strengthens Sobriety

Self-respect acts like a shield against relapse. When you believe you deserve a healthy, stable life, you are less likely to throw it away for a moment of drinking. You will think twice before giving into a craving, because you know the harm it can do to your body and mind. In other words, you protect what you hold dear.

Also, a strong sense of self-respect often goes hand in hand with better relationships. You surround yourself with individuals who value you. That environment, in turn, supports your sobriety. It is a positive cycle: the more you respect yourself, the more you make choices that keep you well, and the better your life becomes overall.

17.17 Conclusion of Chapter 17

Building self-respect is not a quick fix. It unfolds daily as you replace negative thoughts with kinder ones, set boundaries, keep promises, and take pride in small victories. Over time, you shift from seeing yourself as broken by alcohol problems to seeing yourself as a person who made a mistake but learned from it. You become someone who stands up for her own worth.

This transformation does not mean you will never feel doubt or shame again. It means you have the tools to recognize those feelings and address them in a healthier way. By grounding yourself in self-respect, you add another layer of strength to your choice to quit drinking. It bolsters your will, helps you handle stress, and keeps you moving forward.

Chapter 18: Seeing Your Future Without Alcohol

18.1 Introduction: Imagining Tomorrow

Once you have been sober for a while, you might notice something interesting: a new sense of possibility. You are no longer tied to the old habit of drinking. You have extra time, clearer thoughts, and maybe more money in your pocket. The future starts looking different, not simply a repeat of the past. In this chapter, we will explore how to envision a future where alcohol does not control your choices.

A sober future can include many things—better health, stronger relationships, and personal growth. However, it can also seem uncertain. You might worry about challenges that lie ahead. You may wonder if you can stick to this new path when life throws obstacles your way. This chapter provides insights on planning and facing the future with hope, while still staying rooted in the reality of daily life.

18.2 The Benefits of Thinking Ahead

Some people focus only on getting through today without drinking. That is valid in the early stages of quitting. However, as you gain confidence, planning for tomorrow can boost your motivation. It gives you a broader purpose to stay sober. By imagining goals—like improving your career, taking care of your health, or nurturing your family—sobriety becomes the bridge to a life you truly want.

Thinking ahead does not mean you predict everything perfectly. Plans might change. Still, having a general sense of direction allows you to make better decisions now. When you know you want to be financially secure, you will be less tempted to spend money on drinks. When you see yourself living an active lifestyle, you will prioritize healthful activities over alcohol. In short, a clear vision acts like a lighthouse, guiding your daily steps.

18.3 Setting Personal Goals That Inspire You

Seeing the future without alcohol starts by defining what you want in different areas of life. Consider these categories:

1. **Health and Fitness**: Do you want to run a 5K race, lose a certain amount of weight, or simply have more energy to chase your kids around?
2. **Relationships**: Are there strained ties you hope to fix? Do you want to build new friendships that do not revolve around drinking?
3. **Career or Education**: Would you like to start a business, go back to school, or aim for a promotion at work?
4. **Finances**: Do you want to pay off debt, save for a house, or take a special vacation?
5. **Personal Growth**: Is there a skill you have always wanted to learn? A community project you want to start?

Write down one or two goals in each area. Make them specific enough that you can measure progress, but also allow some flexibility in how you achieve them. This balanced approach prevents frustration if you need to adjust along the way.

18.4 Short-Term vs. Long-Term Vision

Goals can be both short-term (like something you want to do in the next 3 to 6 months) and long-term (like where you see yourself in a few years). Short-term goals keep you motivated day to day, while long-term goals give you a bigger picture of why sobriety matters.

For instance, a short-term goal might be to establish a solid morning routine that includes a healthy breakfast and a short exercise session. A long-term goal might be to become a certified yoga instructor, open your own small shop, or move to a new city. By dividing goals into these timelines, you avoid feeling overwhelmed. You have stepping stones that lead to the major vision.

18.5 Facing Fears About the Unknown

When you stop drinking, you may realize you have been using alcohol to hide from certain fears. Perhaps you fear failure, fear success, or fear that you will not fit in without a drink in your hand. Seeing a future without alcohol means acknowledging these fears and deciding to handle them. While it might feel uncomfortable, it is part of stepping into a fuller life.

Try writing down your fears in a notebook. Then, list possible ways to address them. If you fear social rejection, you could join groups that do not center on alcohol, or find friends who support your sober lifestyle. If you fear failing at a new career, break that big goal into small tasks so it seems less daunting. Each step you take to handle fear lessens its power.

18.6 Building Supportive Environments for Your Future

A future free from alcohol is easier to maintain when your surroundings match your intentions. This includes your physical space—like your home being free of alcohol—and also your social circle. Seek out or create situations that uplift you. Maybe that means attending sober meetups, connecting with friends who enjoy hiking or board games, or having family dinners that do not center on wine.

If you stay in settings filled with triggers, you might find it harder to imagine a stable future. This does not mean you must remove yourself from every place that has alcohol; sometimes that is not possible. But you can spend more time in places and with people who accept your sober goals. Over time, these supportive environments shape your day-to-day life, making the idea of returning to old habits less appealing.

18.7 Embracing New Experiences

Once you quit drinking, you may find that your mindset shifts. You might feel braver or more curious. You can handle social situations with a clear head. This can lead you to try things you never would have considered before. Perhaps you decide to learn a second language, join a local club, or take a short trip on your own.

These new experiences can spark excitement and growth. Each time you explore something unfamiliar, you reinforce the idea that life after alcohol is not dull. In fact, it can be richer because you are truly present for each moment. By stepping outside your comfort zone occasionally, you see that challenges can be met, and successes can happen without the crutch of a drink.

18.8 Reconnecting with Loved Ones from a Healthier Place

If alcohol damaged some of your relationships, you may be unsure how to fix them. The future, however, offers room for change. You can reach out to people you might have hurt or neglected. This could mean apologizing for past behavior or simply showing them through consistent actions that you are no longer the person who was trapped by alcohol. Over time, trust can be rebuilt.

In rebuilding ties, you might find that some connections grow even stronger than before, because they are now based on genuine honesty and mutual respect. Others, however, may not fully recover. That can be painful, but it might also open the door to forming new, healthier relationships. Either way, you move forward with a clearer sense of what kind of people you want by your side in the future.

18.9 Protecting Financial Goals and Dreams

Drinking can drain your bank account, whether through bar tabs, liquor store visits, or related medical bills. When you quit, you might notice that your finances are more stable, or at least have the chance to improve. This extra money can be put toward dreams you could not afford before—like taking a course, fixing up your home, or building an emergency fund.

As you plan for the future, consider making a simple budget. List your regular expenses, your income, and what you can save. Give yourself small rewards when you reach certain savings goals. Over time, this responsible approach to money can help you fund bigger dreams, like starting a side business or traveling. Each step you take with your finances solidifies the idea that your sober life can also be more secure.

18.10 Making Time for Personal Reflection

Seeing a life without alcohol also means learning to be at ease with yourself. Alcohol often masks deep feelings or robs you of genuine self-awareness. Now that you are sober, set aside a bit of time—maybe 10 minutes in the evening—to think about the day. What went well? What felt hard? How did you handle stress?

You might do this in a journal or simply in your head. This simple habit helps you track your growth, notice patterns, and keep your future goals in sight. If you find you handled a conflict better than you would have in the past, give yourself credit. If you notice a new worry about the future, plan a step or two to address it. Reflection keeps you connected to your reasons for staying sober and helps you adjust your plans as needed.

18.11 The Role of Hope and Realism

Hope is vital when looking at a future free of alcohol. It gives you the energy to keep going, even when things are tough. However, hope must be balanced with realism. This means understanding that life will still bring stress, sadness, or disappointments at times. Sobriety does not make you immune to hardship; it just helps you face it more effectively.

So, keep your eyes on the good that lies ahead but also stay grounded. If you have a bad day, do not let it erase the hope you have. Remind yourself that setbacks or mistakes do not define the final outcome. You are building a new chapter, and no single event can invalidate all the progress you have made.

18.12 Giving Back: Helping Others on the Same Path

Another way to shape your future is by supporting others who want to quit drinking. This does not mean you have to become a formal counselor, though that is an option. You could simply share your story in a support group, mentor someone who is newer to the process, or volunteer with organizations that help people break free from addiction.

When you give back, you reinforce your own commitment to staying sober. It becomes part of your identity. Plus, it feels rewarding to see someone else benefit from the lessons you have learned. Helping others can also connect you with a positive community of people who share your values. This sense of belonging boosts your motivation and makes the future look brighter, both for you and for those you help.

18.13 Creating a Vision Board or Written Plan

One practical way to keep your future in mind is to create a vision board. This could be a physical board where you pin images that represent your goals and dreams, such as pictures of places you want to visit, skills you want to develop, or quotes that inspire you. If you prefer digital tools, you can make an online collage or a document. The act of collecting these images and words helps solidify what you want.

Alternatively, you can write a short plan that includes bullet points of your goals, steps to reach them, and any deadlines that feel realistic. Review it every now and then, updating your progress or adjusting goals if your interests shift. This keeps you actively involved in shaping your future, rather than passively letting life happen.

18.14 Handling Old Memories That Arise

As you look ahead, old memories of your drinking days might pop up. Some could be painful—like fights you had, things you lost, or times you embarrassed yourself. Others might be oddly tempting, like remembering a night you enjoyed before everything went bad. It is normal for these thoughts to come and go.

When an old memory surfaces, acknowledge it. If it is a painful one, remind yourself that you have learned from that and you are no longer trapped in that behavior. If it is a tempting memory, recall the bigger picture—the morning after, the long-term harm, and why you chose to quit. Let the memory pass without clinging to it. By facing these recollections with honesty, you free yourself from letting them control your future.

18.15 Planning for Big Life Events

Certain events—like weddings, family reunions, or holidays—might still hold a strong link to drinking. Planning ahead is key. If you have a wedding to attend next year, think about how you will manage if they offer champagne to everyone. You can arrange to have a non-alcoholic option in your hand for toasts, or you can step aside when the bar opens.

By considering these details early, you can enjoy big events without feeling anxious. You might bring a friend who understands your choice, or let the host know you need an alternative drink ready. This approach does not have to be dramatic. A simple conversation or a little personal planning can prevent awkward moments and keep you steady on your path.

18.16 Paying Attention to Physical and Mental Health

A future without alcohol can also mean a healthier body and mind. You might notice better sleep, clearer skin, and improved digestion. Mentally, you might experience fewer mood swings or anxiety episodes. Maintaining these improvements means staying aware of your health. Get regular checkups, eat balanced meals, and keep active. If mental health issues appear, do not hesitate to seek help from a professional.

You have already made one major positive change by removing alcohol. By continuing to care for yourself, you ensure that this healthy direction carries on. Over the years, these small but steady actions can significantly raise your overall well-being.

18.17 Conclusion of Chapter 18

Seeing your future without alcohol is both exciting and a bit scary. It is a chance to grow, mend relationships, and explore interests that once seemed out of reach. It also involves facing fears, making plans, and sometimes stepping outside your comfort zone. But remember that sobriety opens doors that were once locked by the habit of drinking.

As you map out goals for health, relationships, finances, and personal growth, your sober life gains direction. You no longer have to define yourself by old mistakes or rely on substances to get through the day. Instead, you can build a life that reflects what you truly care about. Even if you stumble, the vision remains, guiding you forward.

Chapter 19: Helping Other Women

19.1 Introduction: The Value of Shared Support

Once you have come a long way in quitting alcohol, you might notice other women who face similar struggles. Perhaps they are friends, coworkers, neighbors, or even relatives. Many of them may feel alone and afraid to speak up. By offering help, you can make a positive difference in their lives while also solidifying your own choice to stay sober.

This chapter looks at practical ways to help other women who struggle with alcohol. It is not about acting like an expert who has all the answers. Instead, it is about being a caring listener, sharing insights that worked for you, and guiding them toward resources that can help. In return, you often find that helping others strengthens your own resolve. When you see someone else benefit from your experience, it can remind you of how far you have come.

19.2 Recognizing Signs That Someone Needs Support

Sometimes, a woman will openly admit she has a problem. Other times, the signs are subtle. She might make excuses for why she drinks, withdraw from activities she once enjoyed, or speak about constant stress with no relief. Her behavior might change—missing appointments, seeming tired or unfocused, or showing up late to work. You may also hear her make negative remarks about her habits, hinting that she feels stuck.

Recognizing these hints does not mean you should force help on someone. But it may be a chance to gently check in. A simple statement like, "You seem a bit down lately; want to talk?" can open a door. If she brushes you off, you can still let her know you are there if she ever needs a listening ear. The key is to remain approachable without pushing.

19.3 Being a Non-Judgmental Listener

When someone decides to open up, your first job is to listen without judgment. This can be harder than it sounds, especially if you see your own experiences reflected in her words. You might feel tempted to jump in with advice right away or tell her what she "must" do. However, the most crucial step is letting her share. Let her speak without interruption, and avoid making faces or comments that suggest shame or blame.

You can use simple verbal cues like "I see," or "That sounds tough," to show you are listening. If you do not understand something, ask gently: "Could you tell me more about that?" Remember, a woman struggling with alcohol might already carry guilt or fear of judgment. Your open, accepting manner can help her feel safe enough to explore real solutions.

19.4 Sharing Your Own Story Carefully

Telling your own story can be powerful. It shows the other person that she is not alone and that change is possible. However, be mindful not to dominate the conversation with your experiences. The goal is to help her, not to shift all focus onto yourself.

If you choose to share, keep it honest but balanced. Talk about what led you to realize you needed to quit, what early steps you took, and how you felt during the process. If you had slip-ups, mention them briefly to show that imperfection is common. Also, highlight any positive outcomes—like feeling healthier, building better relationships, or having more stability. When you talk about the improvements, do so in a calm, matter-of-fact way, so she sees that a better life is not a fantasy but a real possibility.

19.5 Offering Practical Suggestions and Resources

After listening, you can gently suggest some options that helped you or that you know can help others. This might include:

- **Support Groups**: Local meetings or online communities where people share experiences and advice.
- **Counseling Services**: Therapists or counselors trained in alcohol issues, mental health, or family dynamics.
- **Reading Material**: Books, articles, or trusted websites that explain the science of alcohol dependence and offer tips for quitting.

- **Wellness Activities**: Basic ideas like walking, mild exercise, or journaling to cope with stress rather than reaching for a drink.
- **Budget Tips**: If money problems contribute to her stress, you can share simple budgeting methods or name local financial resources.

Give options without forcing them. She might not be ready to try them all. Even if she is not ready now, knowing these resources exist can ease her sense of isolation. Later, she might pick up one of the suggestions when she feels more prepared to make a change.

19.6 Helping Her Build a Support System

It is one thing to say, "You need a support network," but another to help someone find or create one. You can offer to go with her to a support group meeting if that feels right. If you have a friend who is also sober, you could introduce them. Sometimes, just being available for regular check-ins—like a quick text each morning or a short call—can make a difference.

If she has family members who might be supportive, encourage her to talk openly with them about her decision to cut down or quit drinking. If she is worried about judgment, perhaps she could choose one trusted family member to start with, someone who might understand. The idea is to show her that she does not have to do this alone, and that there are people who can stand by her if she asks.

19.7 Respecting Her Readiness to Change

One key rule is to respect where the other person is in her process. If she is merely curious about cutting back but not fully committed, you can give gentle guidance without pushing for a full stop right away. Pushing too hard can cause her to shut down or avoid you, especially if she is not at that stage of readiness.

On the other hand, if she seems eager to make a big change now, you can offer more direct help—like talking about withdrawal symptoms, finding a counselor, or setting up a plan for handling cravings. Try to match your support to her current mindset, letting her lead the pace. This approach fosters trust and reduces the feeling of being lectured.

19.8 Being Mindful of Your Own Boundaries

Helping others does not mean sacrificing your own well-being. If your friend or acquaintance is in crisis, you can suggest professional help rather than trying to handle everything alone. You might guide her toward hotlines, clinics, or emergency services if she is at serious risk. If you find that supporting someone is triggering your own cravings or stressing you to the point of losing balance, it is okay to step back.

Set clear limits on what you can do. For instance, you might decide to be available for phone calls during the day but not late at night, or you might only meet in neutral, safe places. You can care for someone while still taking care of yourself. In fact, keeping healthy boundaries models responsible behavior and self-respect, which can inspire the person you are trying to help.

19.9 Encouraging Self-Care and Healthy Coping Strategies

Often, women who lean on alcohol do not have enough practical ways to deal with stress or emotional pain. One huge gift you can offer is showing them alternative coping strategies. This might include:

- **Relaxation Techniques**: Simple breathing exercises, short meditation, or calming music.
- **Basic Exercise**: Suggest short walks, gentle stretching, or low-impact routines that fit her schedule.
- **Hobbies**: If she once enjoyed painting, writing, cooking, or other creative activities, encourage her to pick them up again as a stress-reliever.
- **Mindful Moments**: Taking a few quiet minutes each day to check in with feelings rather than suppress them with a drink.

When you share these ideas, keep them simple. Overly complex routines can feel intimidating at first. If you can do a few of these activities with her, it might give her the confidence to keep going on her own.

19.10 Offering Accountability Support

Accountability can be a big help. You might arrange a system where she texts or calls you at certain times—maybe after work, which might be her usual drinking period—to let you know she is staying on track. You can also swap progress notes each day or week. This does not mean you police her actions, but rather that you serve as a friendly checkpoint. Sometimes, just knowing someone will ask can reduce impulses to drink.

In turn, she could help you maintain some of your own positive habits, like exercising regularly or managing stress. It can become a mutual support relationship, which feels less one-sided and more like a team effort.

19.11 Handling a Situation Where She Slips or Relapses

No matter how well-intentioned you are, the person you are helping might slip up and drink again. It is important not to react with harsh criticism or disappointment. Instead, remind her that a slip does not erase all progress. Ask if she wants to talk about what triggered it. Encourage her to return to the methods and routines that helped her before. Suggest updating her plan to avoid the same trigger in the future.

Stay calm and compassionate, but also be clear that she has the power to choose her response next time. If this behavior repeats often, you might suggest more formal treatment, like counseling or an outpatient program. Remember, you cannot fix her problem for her. You can only offer support and information. The decision to keep trying must come from her.

19.12 Sharing Community Resources

Many places have local shelters, community centers, or clinics that offer help for those battling alcohol misuse. As someone who has found your own path to sobriety, you might have knowledge of these resources. You could share the phone numbers, addresses, or website links. You could also mention any free or low-cost programs for women in particular. Some churches or nonprofit groups host group sessions where women can safely discuss addiction and related challenges.

If you are in an online community, you can pass along links to supportive forums or websites that talk about quitting alcohol in a caring manner. The more options you provide, the more likely she is to find something that fits her style and comfort level.

19.13 Being an Example of a Sober Lifestyle

One of the best ways to help other women is by living out the changes yourself. When they see that you can enjoy social events without alcohol, handle stress by non-alcoholic means, and maintain a healthy routine, it shows them that sober living can be real and not just theory. You do not have to pretend to be perfect—sharing that you still face temptations or have rough days can make you more relatable. But you can also show that you keep going, keep using your methods, and keep protecting your well-being.

This example might inspire them more than any words alone. Actions speak loudly. A woman might think, "If she can do it, maybe I can too." That spark can be the start of a genuine effort on her part.

19.14 Avoiding the Role of "Fixer" or "Savior"

It is easy to slip into a pattern of trying to rescue someone. But in the end, each person must decide to change for her own reasons. If you push too hard or try to control her entire recovery process, you risk damaging the connection and exhausting yourself. You might end up feeling resentment if she does not follow your advice. On her side, she might feel smothered or judged.

Instead, see yourself as a guide or companion. Offer information, share your own experiences, listen, and encourage. Let her know you believe in her ability to make decisions. Doing so respects her dignity and can lead to a healthier dynamic, both for her and for you.

19.15 Handling Emotional Strain as a Helper

Supporting someone who is dealing with alcohol problems can be stressful. You might feel anxious, worried, or even take on their sadness as your own. If you notice that this strain is growing, take steps to care for yourself. Confide in a close friend or counselor about how you feel. Make sure you continue any self-care routines you rely on—like exercise, journaling, or quiet time.

It is also okay to set limits if the other person's crisis is consuming too much of your time or emotional energy. You can politely explain that you are there for them, but they might need additional professional help or a wider support network. Remember, you cannot pour from an empty cup. Tending to your own needs makes you a stronger ally for someone else.

19.16 When Your Support May Not Be Enough

Sometimes, despite your best efforts, the woman you want to help may not show real progress. She might continue to drink heavily or push you away. You may have to accept that your role is limited. Continue to express concern, but recognize that you cannot force change. Let her know you are willing to help if she decides to seek it, but keep your own boundaries firm.

If her drinking poses a direct danger (for instance, driving under the influence or putting children at risk), you might need to involve professionals or authorities. This step is tough, but sometimes necessary to protect her safety or the safety of others. Such a move does not mean you have given up on her; it shows you care about well-being in the broader sense.

19.17 Conclusion of Chapter 19

Helping other women who struggle with alcohol can be rewarding and challenging at the same time. Your own journey without alcohol can serve as a source of hope and practical knowledge. By listening without judgment, sharing resources, and respecting each person's readiness to change, you can be a positive force in someone's life.

Remember, you are not responsible for someone else's recovery. All you can do is offer genuine support, encouragement, and reliable information. Ultimately, each individual must choose her own path. Still, the care and understanding you provide can make a world of difference, especially for someone who feels lost or alone. Along the way, you might find your own dedication to sobriety growing stronger. There is something powerful about guiding others. It can remind you why your own health and freedom matter so much.

In the next and final chapter, we will explore how to keep your progress strong over the long haul. We will discuss practical ways to watch for old triggers, stay inspired, and live in a way that protects all the gains you have made.

Chapter 20: Keeping Your Progress Strong

20.1 Introduction: A Life-Long Commitment

Reaching a stable place in your sobriety is a significant achievement. Yet, stopping alcohol for a few months or even a year is just one stage. The real goal is to keep those gains strong and continue living free from the pull of old habits. This means staying alert, caring for your mental and physical health, and regularly checking in with yourself.

In this final chapter, we will look at how to maintain your progress for the long term. We will cover methods to handle ongoing triggers, how to remain motivated even when life changes, and practical tips for ensuring you do not slip back into the cycle of drinking. These strategies can help you settle into a lifestyle where alcohol no longer has a hold on you.

20.2 Regular Self-Checkups

One of the best ways to keep your progress is to stay aware of how you feel mentally and emotionally. Schedule regular self-checkups—this could be once a week, once a month, or whenever you sense a shift in your mindset. Ask yourself questions like:

- **Am I feeling more stressed than usual?**
- **Have I noticed any new cravings or urges?**
- **Have I neglected any healthy routines—like exercise, balanced meals, or support meetings?**
- **Am I spending time with people or in places that tempt me to drink?**

By checking in with yourself, you catch small problems before they grow. If you see a red flag, act right away—return to a healthy routine, call a friend, or schedule a counseling session if needed. Quick action can prevent a minor slump from turning into a major setback.

20.3 Using a Balanced Lifestyle as a Shield

Keeping your sober life requires a broader sense of balance in daily living. This includes:

1. **Healthy Eating**: A good diet helps stabilize energy and mood. If you skip meals, blood sugar swings can worsen cravings or heighten stress.
2. **Consistent Sleep**: Aim for a regular bedtime. Lack of rest can make you irritable, undermine motivation, and wear down your resolve.
3. **Physical Activity**: This does not have to mean intense workouts. Even short walks or gentle stretching helps clear the mind and release tension.
4. **Meaningful Hobbies**: Leisure activities that spark your interest can keep you fulfilled. A hobby distracts from cravings and builds self-esteem.
5. **Social Connections**: Spending time with people who respect your decision reinforces it. Avoid or limit contact with those who push you to drink.

Combining these habits forms a sturdy foundation. When you feel balanced in your body and mind, you are less likely to seek escapes in alcohol.

20.4 Handling Shifts in Your Life Situation

Over time, life changes. You might move to a new city, start a different job, or go through relationship transitions. Such shifts can disrupt familiar routines. If your support group or counselor was local, a move could make you lose that resource. Or a new job might come with added stress. If you are not careful, these changes can weaken your resolve.

Plan for big changes as best you can. Before you move, look up support groups in your new area. If you change jobs, consider how you will manage potential after-work social events. By thinking ahead, you avoid being caught off guard. If life surprises you, take a moment to breathe and adapt your sobriety plan to your new circumstances. Remind yourself that the principles remain the same, even if your setting is different.

20.5 Keeping Inspiration Alive

Early in your sober journey, you might feel strong motivation—like relief from hangovers, improved health, or pride in reaching new milestones. Over time, that excitement can fade as the novelty wears off. It is important to renew your sense of purpose. One way is to keep a journal of daily or weekly reflections about what you are gaining by staying sober. You could note your improved energy levels, better mood, or money saved.

You might also set fresh goals, even small ones, to keep yourself engaged. If you have never tried hiking, for example, see if you can tackle a local trail. If you have always dreamed of painting, sign up for a beginner's class. Achievements in new areas can provide the boost that once came from the early excitement of quitting alcohol.

20.6 Keeping a Circle of Support

Though you may feel stable, it is wise to maintain a network of supportive people. These could be sober friends, accountability buddies, counselors, or trusted family members. Keep in touch, whether through calls, texts, or in-person meetups. If you used to attend a support group, consider dropping by now and then, even if you no longer feel it is essential every week. You might be able to help someone else, and it also keeps you in tune with your own progress.

Let your friends and family know that even though you are doing well, you still value their encouragement. You can share updates about how you are handling life without alcohol. These connections can catch small warning signs you might miss. For instance, a close friend may notice if you start withdrawing socially or showing signs of stress.

20.7 Revisiting Old Lessons

Sometimes, going back to the basics is a good idea. Re-read parts of this book or any other resources that helped you. Remind yourself of the triggers you identified early on, the coping strategies you used, and the reasons you quit drinking. Overconfidence can sneak in, leading you to think you no longer need those tactics. A quick review can ground you and keep those tools at the forefront of your mind.

If you wrote a personal plan at the beginning—like listing your triggers, resources, and motivations—check it again. Update it if anything has changed. Add new insights you have gained along the way. Treat it as a living document that grows with you, rather than something you wrote and forgot.

20.8 Watching Out for Subtle Warning Signs

Cravings do not always show up as strong, urgent desires to drink. Sometimes, they are more subtle. You might catch yourself thinking, "I deserve a little fun," or "A small drink will not hurt me." Or you might daydream about the "good old times," ignoring the negative parts. These quiet signals can be tricky.

When you notice these thoughts, do not panic. Acknowledge them and remind yourself why you quit. Think of the bigger picture—the stress, the health issues, the financial problems, or the emotional turmoil that alcohol caused. Then, shift your attention to something constructive. This could be a short walk, a chat with a friend, or a quick activity you enjoy. By taking these subtle signs seriously, you stop them from growing into full-blown cravings.

20.9 Keeping Up with Healthy Boundaries

As life moves on, it is easy to let old boundaries slip. Maybe you start hanging out with friends who drink heavily again or spending time in bars out of curiosity. Being confident in your sobriety does not mean exposing yourself unnecessarily to risky situations. Check in: Are you regularly putting yourself in environments where alcohol is the main focus? If so, why?

While you do not have to avoid every place that serves drinks, you can still limit your time there or bring a sober friend along. Boundaries are not just about physical spaces. They also apply to emotional limits, like saying "no" to events that could overwhelm you with pressure to drink, or refusing to store alcohol in your home. Keep these boundaries firm as part of your long-term plan.

20.10 Learning from Others' Experiences

Staying sober is a journey that countless people have taken. You can benefit from the collective wisdom out there. Reading stories of women who have stayed sober for many years can be uplifting. Hearing about their setbacks, solutions, and triumphs can remind you that you are not alone. Some might suggest new coping tools you have not tried.

You could also look into podcasts or online communities where people discuss maintaining sobriety over the long haul. Stay open to fresh ideas. Even if you think you have everything figured out, there is always something new to learn from another person's viewpoint. This ongoing learning helps you adapt to life's changes.

20.11 Giving Yourself Time to Grow

Sobriety is not a race. Sometimes, women feel frustrated if they do not achieve major life changes quickly. You might see someone else who quit drinking and then seemed to climb the career ladder or fix their marriage right away. Remember that each person's path is unique. It may take longer for you to feel fully stable or to fix certain problems. That is normal.

Be patient. Focus on small daily improvements. If your life is much calmer now than it was a year ago, that is progress. If you handle conflicts better or have improved your finances, that is progress, too. Recognize these gains, no matter how small, instead of obsessing over perfection. Each steady step forward beats rushing and risking a setback.

20.12 Preparing for Unexpected Stress

Life can throw surprises—illness, job loss, family emergencies, or personal grief. These events can test your sobriety because they bring intense stress or sadness. One way to prepare is to keep a mini emergency plan in mind. Ask yourself: "If something truly upsetting happens, who can I call? What immediate step can I take instead of drinking?"

This might be a quick breathing exercise, a phone call to your accountability buddy, or a short walk to clear your head. You might also keep a small list of encouraging reminders in your wallet or phone. That list could include reasons you quit, phone numbers of supportive contacts, or brief statements like, "This feeling will pass, and I do not want to throw away all I have gained." By being ready, you reduce the power of sudden stress.

20.13 Accepting That Life Is Not Always Perfect

One hidden trap is thinking that quitting alcohol will solve every problem. While sobriety often leads to better health, improved relationships, and more clarity, life still has problems. You might have to handle everyday issues, personality conflicts, or financial worries. Accepting this fact keeps you from feeling disillusioned when normal life troubles arise.

Remind yourself that being sober does not mean you must be happy 24/7. It means you face challenges with a clear mind, and you do not add the extra burden of alcohol-induced harm. By staying realistic, you spare yourself the disappointment of expecting a life without flaws. Instead, you learn to handle ups and downs in a healthier way.

20.14 Ongoing Therapy or Group Support (If Needed)

You may decide you do not need constant therapy or weekly support meetings forever. However, keeping a connection to these resources can be a safety net. Some women continue meeting with a counselor monthly or attend a group once a month to check in. It is a way to measure progress, address new issues, and maintain accountability.

If you find life is going smoothly, you might skip sessions for a while. Just remember that it is okay to return if you sense old feelings surfacing. Therapy or group meetings are not a sign of weakness. They are tools that help you grow stronger and keep your foot on solid ground.

20.15 Sharing Your Knowledge with Others

As you move forward, you might naturally find ways to support other women—like we discussed in Chapter 19. By continuing to share what you have learned, you keep the lessons fresh in your mind. You also build a community of caring. Some women choose to volunteer in local programs or mentor newcomers in a support group. Others just keep an open door for friends who are curious about sober living.

This sharing also helps you reflect on your journey. Each time you explain why you quit or how you handle cravings, you reaffirm your own commitment. You might even learn new tips from those you mentor because they bring their own ideas to the table.

20.16 Celebrating Milestones

While we avoid certain words, marking milestones in a positive way remains important. You can note each year of sobriety with a simple personal ritual—like writing a letter to yourself about how you have grown, or planning a day trip to a place that symbolizes freedom to you. It does not have to be fancy or public. The point is to recognize the effort and progress you have made.

If you have people who supported you, you can share your milestone with them. Let them know how their help mattered. Such moments build confidence for the next stage of life. They show that time is passing in a good way, without the chaos of alcohol overshadowing your achievements.

20.17 Conclusion of Chapter 20

Keeping your progress strong is a long-term endeavor, but it does not have to be burdensome. By practicing regular self-checkups, staying mindful of boundaries, nurturing a balanced lifestyle, and revisiting the basic lessons that led you here, you can safeguard your sobriety. As life evolves, you adapt your plan, remain open to support, and continue to set new goals that bring purpose and joy.

Sobriety is not a single victory; it is a continuing path of growth. Over time, you may find that the thought of returning to old habits feels distant because you are too invested in the healthier, freer life you have built. You see that challenges come and go, but they can be met without numbing yourself with a drink. This realization forms the bedrock of a life lived on your own terms.

Final Thoughts

With all 20 chapters covered, you have an in-depth guide that addresses many parts of quitting alcohol, from the earliest realizations to helping others and maintaining your freedom for years to come. Each chapter offers practical methods, simple language, and a step-by-step approach to building a stable foundation.

www.ingramcontent.com/pod-product-compliance
Lightning Source LLC
LaVergne TN
LVHW012109070526
838202LV00056B/5681